Super
Foods
BOOK

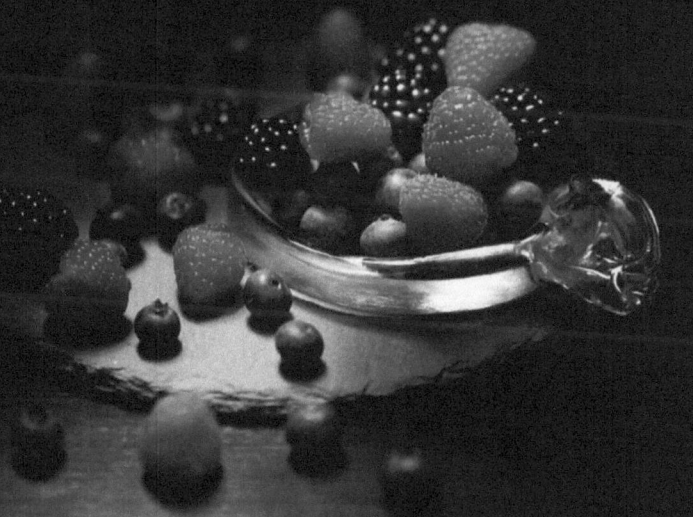

Barbara Nichols

DISCLAIMER

These statements have not been evaluated by the Food and Drug Administration (FDA). The products mentioned on this site are not intended to diagnose, treat, cure or prevent any disease. Note that the contents here are not presented by a medical practitioner, and that any and all health care planning should be made under the guidance of your own medical and health practitioners. The content within only presents an overview based upon research for educational purposes and does not replace medical advice from a practicing physician. Further, the information in this manual is provided "as is" and without warranties of any kind either expressed or implied. Under no circumstances, including, but not limited to, negligence, shall the seller/DISTRIBUTOR OF THIS INFORMATION BE LIABLE FOR ANY SPECIAL OR CONSEQUENTIAL DAMAGES THAT RESULT FROM THE USE OF, OR THE INABILITY TO USE, THE INFORMATION PRESENTED HERE. DO NOT FOLLOW THE INFORMATION IN THIS BOOK IF YOU ARE PREGNANT OR NURSING

Content

INTRODUCTION

You've probably experienced this: The media or some expert on Facebook tells you to eat this to stay healthy, or to eat this to lose weight.

Then the very next day there are conflicting reports telling us to stay away from those foods.

What's an eater to do?

Well, thankfully, many doctors, scientists and nutrition experts have reached the same conclusion about a group of foods which are considered superior to all the rest—they're known as Superfoods.

No, this isn't a marketing gimmick from a big food maker. This is real science with real results that can change your life!

To give you an idea, if "normal" people were like "normal" food, Superfoods would be like Spider-Man or Wonder Woman.

They have all these amazing nutrients and properties that scientists have discovered can help lower your cholesterol, keep your brain sharp, help you lose weight, keep you looking young, and even help protect us from cancer!

Seriously, Superfoods rock!

These foods are loaded with so many nutrients that eating them can have a demonstrable effect over the course of your life. These are validated in scientific study after study.

Each Superfood helps you in different ways. You have to know which special properties each one possesses so you know what they can do for you.

The great thing about most Superfoods is that you can find them in your grocery store.

To get the most value out of these foods, you should not overcook them. Heat will oxidize many of the nutrients. Applying a little heat is OK, just don't overdo it.

Most importantly, enjoy the food and know that you're improving the health of you and and the people you feed!

This book is broken down into two parts:

First, we'll go over individual Superfoods. You'll learn about each food and its health benefits.

In the second part of the book, we'll talk about how you can achieve specific health goals with Superfoods.

Let's get started...

PART 1

SUPER FOODS

ACAI BERRY

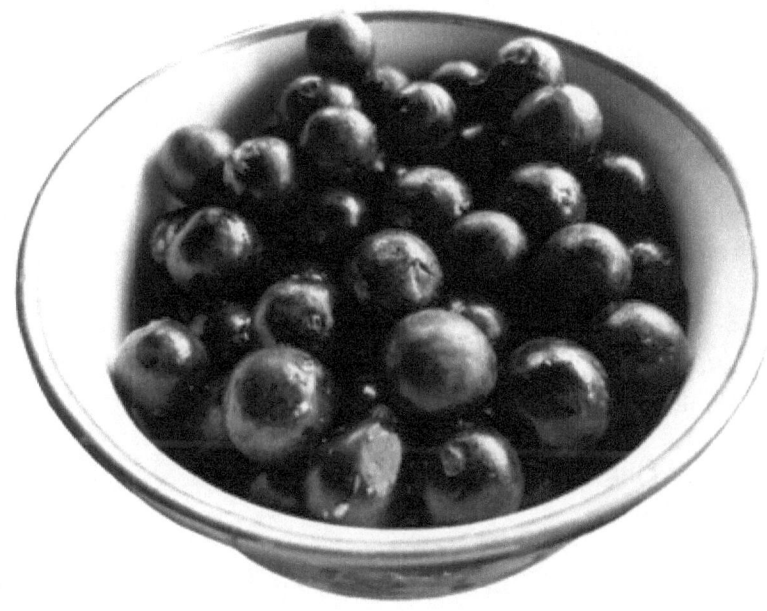

The acai berry from the Amazonian floodplains has long been used by the natives in Brazil for increased energy and maintaining overall health.

Recently, the rest of the world has started using Acai for anti-aging.

This dark purple palm fruit, the size of a blueberry, has been shown to have tremendous health enhancing powers found in its antioxidant-rich, dark purple pulp.

Acai lets you enjoy many of the heart health benefits of wine without the side effects of alcohol.

The world is just beginning to discover this small, wonder berry's health promoting, curative properties and its benefits for health and beauty.

The acai berry, pronounced ah-sigh-ee in Portuguese, is the fruit of the palm tree Euterpe oleracea that grows naturally all over Brazil, in the rain forests of the Amazon plains.

The fruits grow in large clusters between the palm's ribbon-like leaves.

The thin layer of edible, purple pulp around a large seed has long been used by natives for skin and digestive disorders.

The ripe berries which are a rich dark purple are hand harvested. Typically, the pulp is quickly separated and frozen to preserve all its nutritional properties.

Research into the acai berry has found it to be power-packed with healthy goodness.

The acai berries have been found to contain extremely high concentrations of the potent antioxidant flavonoids called anthocyanins, also found in red wine and known to help lower cholesterol levels, protect blood vessels, reduce inflammation, fight cancer cells and provide immediate energy.

South American locals also refer to acai as natures Viagra!

Acai also provides proteins and fiber and contains the fatty acids omega-6 and omega-9 in addition to essential amino acids.

This miracle berry has been gaining in popularity due to these health-enhancing properties.

Health buffs, natural cure seekers and athlete seeking a performance edge have finally found a new, single source for concentrated vitamins and antioxidants, fiber and protein, fatty acids and minerals.

Are you getting excited about everything this berry can do for you?

There's still more...

Acai increases stamina, improves circulation thus improving mental focus, reduces cholesterol, and improves digestion.

Its antioxidant properties are greater than those of grapes, olives, red wine, and other plant products.

Acai is already found in specialty and organic grocery stores, whole food retailers, and health food stores. Many chain stores are stocking acai berry products as pure frozen juice and pure frozen pulp.

In addition, several Internet sites offer good quality products.

It is very important to buy acai berry products from reliable sources so that there has been no loss of nutrients due to delays in processing or storage. Unreliable sources could sell low-quality products which have lost their vitamin and antioxidant properties due to freezing delays or improper harvesting.

The Amazonian farmers have long worked with these berries and continue to traditionally harvest, package and quickly freeze the berries so that all the nutritional benefits and fabulous taste are preserved.

Today they share their secret miracle with the rest of the world.

Acai Berry Summary

• Acai lets you enjoy many of the heart health benefits of wine without the side effects of alcohol.

• The thin layer of edible, purple pulp around a large seed has long been used by natives for skin and digestive disorders.

• The acai berries have been found to contain extremely high concentrations of the potent antioxidant flavonoids called anthocyanins, also found in red wine and known to help lower cholesterol levels, protect blood vessels, reduceinflammation, fight cancer cells and provide immediate energy.

• South American locals also refer to acai as natures Viagra!

• Acai increases stamina, improves circulation thus improving mental focus, reduces cholesterol, and improves digestion.

WOLFBERRY

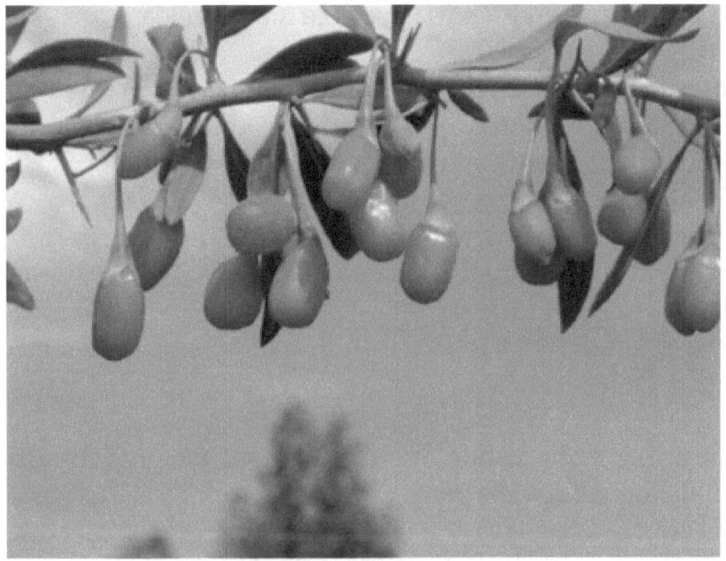

Used in Chinese Medicine as far back as 1000 ad. **Wolfberries help strengthen your immune system, treat diabetes, and lower high blood pressure.**

Wolfberries grow on bushes in the wild between April and October in the North West region of China.

The harvesting of the fruit is done from June to October.

The growth of the wolfberry is dependent on the local conditions and weather. It comes in an oblong shape, is delicious to eat, and when it is ready to be picked it turns a lovely red color.

Science has named the primary agent that is active in the fruit as Lycium Barbarum Polysaccharide or LBP for short.

The amount of LBP is dependent on the berry itself with the highest LBP found in better quality berries.

It has 21 trace minerals and 19 types of amino acids.

An interesting fact is that Wolfberries have more vitamin C than an orange, more beta carotene than a carrot and a protein content that is almost equivalent to bee pollen.

The Chinese have grown Wolfberries from as far back as the Tang dynasty, which ruled from 1000 to 1400 AD.

One can find reference to this fruit in traditional Chinese medical books.

The most important feature of this fruit is the fact that it nourishes the yin factor and not the yang.

Yin and yang are the two forces that the Chinese believe are part of the human system, with yin being the material part and yang standing for energy and function.

So the fruit actually treats the body holistically.

Now the world is fast getting educated about the health benefits of the wolfberry.

The wolfberry belongs to the family of the Solanaceae plant family.

It is used mostly in teas, stews, soups, and wine. The fruit may be eaten raw as well.

There has been a lot of research by the modern world to ascertain the usefulness of this fruit and these studies have only confirmed what the ancients maintained.

Some of the ways wolfberry works its magic are its ability to nourish the blood, strengthen the eyes, the kidneys and the liver.

These in turn help you with problems like fatigue, insomnia, eyesight problems, hearing problems, liver disease, headaches, and dizziness to name a few.

This fruit is seen in many herbal preparations and is generally considered a tonic for overall good health.

It also has antioxidant and anti-aging properties.

So, if you are looking for overall health benefits and some way to give your system a boost, try out the wolfberry. It has a lot of benefits which can pep you up and make you feel good.

Wolfberry Summary

●Wolfberries help strengthen your immune system, treat diabetes, and lower high blood pressure.

●An interesting fact is that Wolfberries have more vitamin C than an orange, more beta carotene than a carrot and a protein content that is almost equivalent to bee pollen.

●Some of the ways wolfberry works its magic are its ability to nourish the blood, strengthen the eyes, the kidneys and the liver.

•Helps you with problems like fatigue, insomnia, eyesight problems, hearing problems, liver disease, headaches, and dizziness to name a few.

•It also has antioxidant and anti-aging properties.

POMEGRANATE

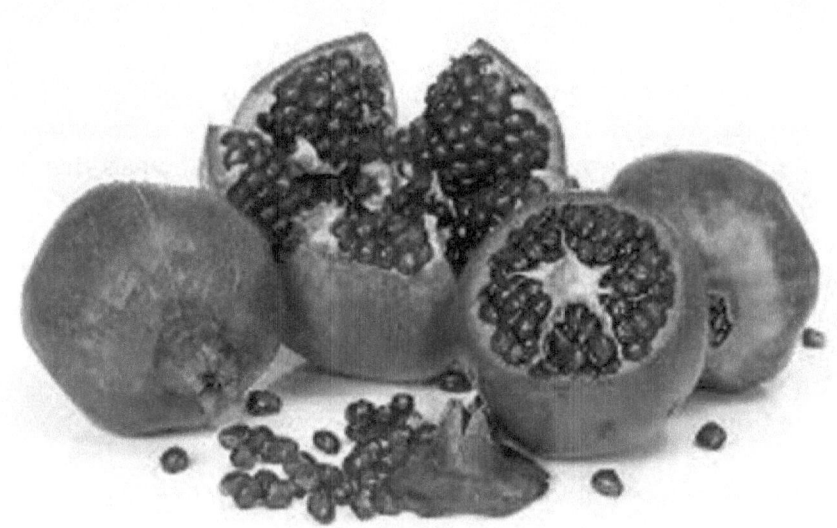

In ancient times pomegranates were called the "fertility fruit" - today they're used to treat sore throats, rheumatism, and inflammation.

Only recently have scientists begun to investigate the health benefits of the pomegranate.

Recent studies have stated that pomegranate juice contains three times the amount of antioxidants as found in red wine and green tea.

Besides this, the pomegranate also contains other important minerals such as potassium and important vitamins such as niacin and Vitamin C in substantial quantities.

Pomegranates also have fiber in significant amounts.

What has the pomegranate traditionally been used for?

It has been a popular folk medicine in India, Iran and throughout the Middle East and other places where it is abundantly available.

The skin of the pomegranate is rather tough and is either brownish or dark red in color. It is approximately the same size as an orange or apple. The juicy red pulp of the pomegranate is the part that is edible.

Let's take a look at the pomegranates history.

The name pomegranate has its origins in a Latin term, which is used to indicate 'fruit of many seeds'. The name is well deserved as the fruit has an abundance of seeds within its tough rind.

Ancient Egyptian folklore, as well as Greek mythology has many references to this fruit, which was strongly associated with fertility.

As everybody knows, eating a pomegranate could be a laborious process.

The hundreds of seeds are encased in a bitter membrane. Taking off this bitter membrane is what can take a long time as it leaves a not-so-good taste in the mouth if eaten.

Pomegranates are available in different varieties all over the world.

The best way to distinguish between the different types is by checking the color of the seeds. Pomegranate seeds could be dark pink, light red and sometimes a deep scarlet color.

The best pomegranates to buy are those that have the deepest color and feel heavy. The skin should feel moist and smooth, not dry and cracked.

Pomegranates can be kept for two to three days at room temperature and will stay fresh up to three months in the refrigerator.

Pomegranates typically contain about 100 calories, which makes them a fruit of choice for dieters.

Pomegranate juice is another great way to enjoy this delicious fruit.

Pomegranate juice is used to enhance the taste of a variety of dishes including vinaigrettes, marinades, sauces, and jellies.

Many people love to sprinkle pomegranate seeds over their desserts or salads for that extra zing. Garnishing poultry, fish and meats with pomegranate seeds enhances the flavor of the dish.

The pomegranate season does not last for too long so make the best of it while you can. You are sure to enjoy the delicious taste and of course the multitude of health benefits that come your way.

Pomegranate Summary

•In ancient times pomegranates were called the "fertility fruit" - today they're used to treat sore throats, rheumatism, and inflammation.

•Besides this, the pomegranate also contains other important minerals such as potassium and important vitamins such as niacin and Vitamin C in substantial quantities.

ORANGES

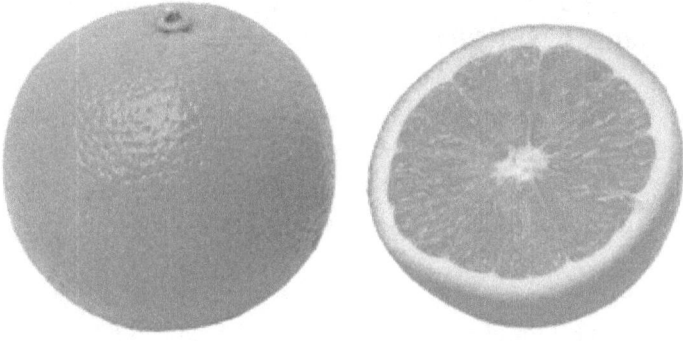

If you're not familiar with carotenoids you soon will be because carotenoids have shown incredible promise in fighting many types of cancer.

Oranges have more than 20 compounds in the carotenoid family.

Oranges in any form are great - be it the fruit, the fresh juice, the packaged juice, the jams, the jellies, the marmalade, salad dressings, and desserts.

The orange is part of the citrus fruit family and all of them are oh, so healthy for us.

Throughout the ages, citrus fruits have been used for their taste, flavor and nutritional value. The fact that they are said to add years to your life when eaten on a regular basis is, of course, an added benefit.

The main healthy ingredient in oranges is vitamin C.

However, that's not all there is to the orange.

Oranges are power-packed with more, lots more. It's got 170 phytochemicals, with 20 carotenoid compounds.

Also present are limonoids which impart that slightly bitter, tangy taste to all citrus fruits.

These are also thought to be cancer-fighters and the orange is a rich source.

The best-known fact about the orange is its vitamin C content.

Being loaded with vitamin C is what elevates oranges to Superfood status.

Just one orange, and an average-sized one at that could give you over 90% of your daily requirement of vitamin C.

So it pays to eat or drink up your oranges so you stay fit.

What exactly does vitamin C do to make it such an important asset as far as health goes?

Well, it is basically a fighter.

If you can get a big dose of vitamin C in your body at the very start of a cold or flu you can sometimes stop it. At the very least it will minimize the effects.

Vitamin C is a great antioxidant as well as an essential nutrient.

Vitamin C is water soluble and is known to repair the cell damage done by the free radicals in the body. It is also known to be one of the best substances to strengthen your immune system.

This vitamin is vital in keeping the immune system functioning perfectly so this is why it has the reputation of preventing colds and acts as a deterrent to disease invading the body.

The ideal way to take in vitamin C is through your diet rather than just popping pills.

When you eat the orange or drink its juice, you are getting a lot more than just the vitamin C content in the fruit.

You are also getting all that goodness that helps keep you free from disease and the substances that fight disease when it does strike.

Oranges Summary

• The main healthy ingredient in oranges is vitamin C.

• Oranges are power-packed with more, lots more. It's got 170 phytochemicals, with 20 carotenoid compounds.

• Just one orange, and an average-sized one at that could give you over 90% of your daily requirement of vitamin C.

• If you can get a big dose of vitamin C in your body at the very start of a cold or flu you can sometimes stop it. At the very least it will minimize the effects.

•Vitamin C is water soluble and is known to repair the cell damage done by the free radicals in the body. It is also known to be one of the best substances to strengthen your immune system.

GOJI BERRY

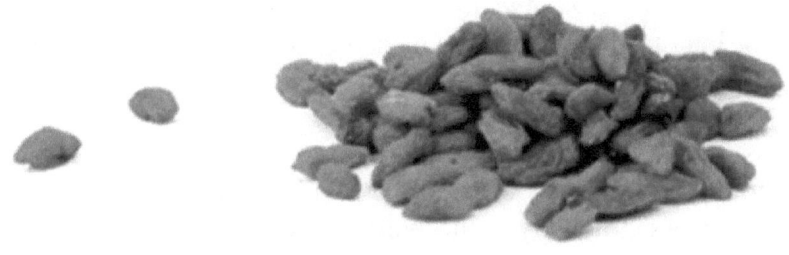

This tiny red fruit from the Himalayas grows in a harsh environment and earned its Superfood status for its anti-aging abilities.

The secret is a special compound scientists call "master molecules" that have the ability to control elements of your body and immune system.

With the number of anti-aging supplements on the market and the variety of foods that lay claim to preserving youth, it is evident that people are more passionate than ever about staying young.

Anti-aging abilities are a big reason the goji berry is gaining in popularity.

The goji berry, bearing the botanical name Lycium barbarum, grows on a vine. The fruit is characteristically small and red and found in abundance in the Himalayan region.

For generations, this fruit has been used in the preparation of medicines.

At one time the benefit of this fruit was a closely guarded secret. The rest of the world discovered the goji berry only recently and since then, they cannot have enough of it!

The Tibetans, Chinese and Indians living in the Himalayas, who have for long been practitioners of herbal medicine, found that the goji berry had the power to heal.

Visitors to this mountainous region carried goji berries back to their homes and thus the word of the goji berry spread, first to the rest of Asia and gradually to the Western world.

Today, the goji berry has various strains and it grows in different parts of the world.

Farmers have taken to cultivating this crop as they have realized its financial benefits. However, the most efficacious fruit still grow in the Himalayan valleys, so when goji supplements are bought it is advisable to verify the source.

Goji berries of the Himalayas are known to have the highest nutritional value and are rich in phytonutrient compounds comprising four polysaccharides, or master molecules as scientists prefer to call them. These master molecules are important for the efficient working of the immune system.

The goji berry can be eaten off the vine or made into juice or supplements, all of which are readily available at supermarkets, specialty stores, or at any food outlet.

Goji Berry Summary

•Anti-aging abilities are a big reason the goji berry is gaining in popularity.

•Goji berries of the Himalayas are known to have the highest nutritional value and are rich in phytonutrient compounds comprising four polysaccharides, or master molecules as scientists prefer to call them. These master molecules are important for the efficient working of the immune system.

SPINACH

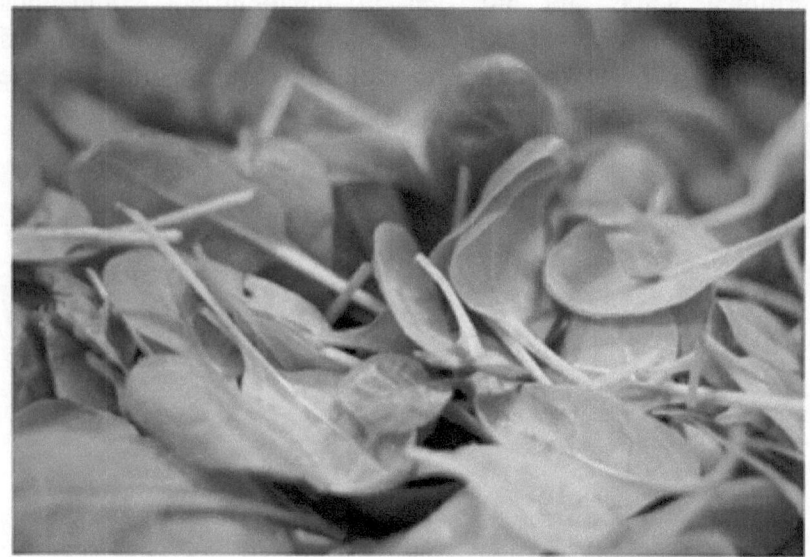

Popeye knew what he was talking about. Eating Spinach is thought to make you stronger, but there are many other reasons you should add this Superfood to your diet.

Nutritionists have for a very long time, considered vegetables that are dark green and leafy to be very healthy when compared to other foods.

Spinach is rich in vitamin C, calcium and beta-carotene.

Spinach is not only full of nutrients, but it's rich in insoluble fiber.

The insoluble fiber that is present in spinach is very good for health, especially the heart.

Spinach not only protects from heart diseases but also brings down the risk of different kinds of cancer, including lung cancer.

Spinach is a rich source of Vitamin K that helps fight cancer-causing substances.

Eye issues like Cataracts are another problem that can be prevented by the consumption of spinach thanks to its high content of beta-carotene.

Vegetables that have dark green leaves like kale and spinach are very good for overall health.

Spinach contains carotenoids, like beta-carotene, which are very strong antioxidants that help in the protection against many health problems.

Eating spinach can also help control homocysteine levels in the blood.

A diet that is rich in beta-carotene, folic acid and vitamin C is an easy way to bring down the levels of homocysteine in the blood.

A common problem among older people is macular degeneration.

Spinach and other leafy vegetables are very helpful as they alleviate macular degeneration-related risk factors.

Spinach is easily available and is not very expensive.

It can be bought at any supermarket, grocery store or at any local market. Spinach is also available in other varieties like such as powdered spinach and canned spinach.

You could use these if you are unable to find fresh spinach, but one thing to remember is that fresh spinach is always better.

Spinach Summary

●Spinach is is rich in vitamin C, calcium and beta-carotene.

●The insoluble fiber that is present in spinach is very good for health, especially the heart.

●Spinach is a rich source of Vitamin K that helps fight cancer-causing substances.

●Eye issues like cataract are another problem that can be prevented by the consumption of spinach thanks to its high content of beta-carotene.

●Eating spinach can also help control homocysteine levels in the blood.

GREEN TEA

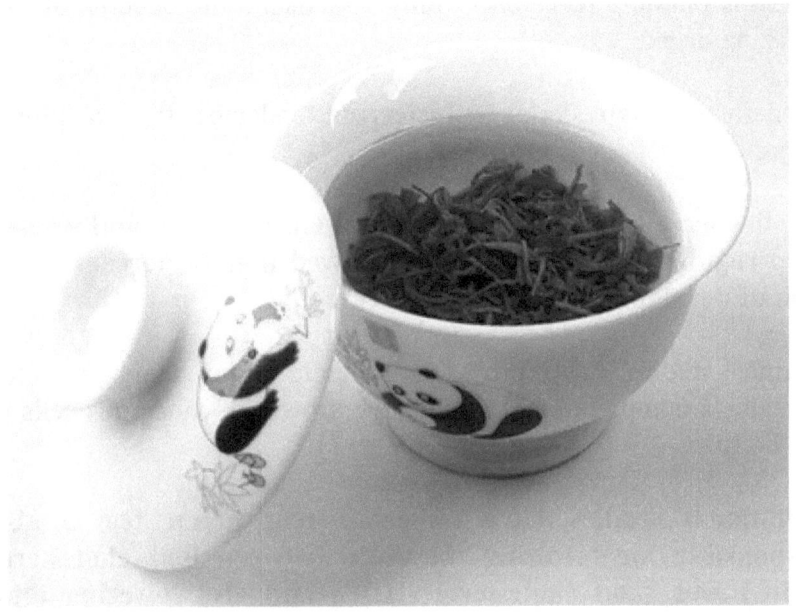

By the year 780 ad. the preparation of Green Tea was considered a fine art.

It's been used to treat everything from headaches, insomnia, and digestive problems. Most recently it's been looked at to help cure cancer.

The health benefits of green tea are well documented.

The Chinese, renowned for their knowledge of ancient herbal medicines, have always known and believed in the curative properties of green tea.

Since ancient times the Chinese have used green tea as a traditional medicine in the treatment of a wide range of ailments ranging from depression and insomnia to stomachaches and headaches.

There is ongoing research to fully understand the benefits of this amazing drink.

Modern research done by scientists endorses the traditional curative properties of green tea.

Studies have consistently shown that Chinese men and women who regularly drank green tea showed a sixty percent lower risk of developing esophageal cancer.

Further studies have provided concrete proof that green tea contains a compound that inhibits the growth of cancerous cells in the body.

Additional studies have indicated that green tea is also responsible for lowering the ratio between bad cholesterol (LDL) and good cholesterol (HDL) and also lowering total cholesterol levels in the body.

Green tea is considered an effective cure for high cholesterol levels, lowered immune system function, cancer, infections, high blood pressure, cardiovascular problems, and rheumatoid arthritis.

The magic of green tea seems to be the fact that it is very high in polyphenols, of which the most significant is epigallocatechin gallate (EGCG).

This powerful antioxidant is responsible for inhibiting the growth of cancer cells.

EGCG has the ability to kill cancer cells in the body without causing any injury to the healthy tissue.

EGCG also has the capacity to lower bad cholesterol (LDL) levels and helps to prevent the formation of blood clots.

This is one of the possible reasons that green tea has been so effective in preventing strokes and heart disease.

Recent studies have proven that EGCG is two times as powerful as resveratrol, an ingredient in red wine that is known to counter the ill effects of a high-fat diet.

What makes green tea so special?

Though many teas are sourced from the leaves of the camellia sinensis plant, the difference between green tea and the other varieties of tea lies in the method of processing.

Green tea leaves are steamed and this helps prevent the critical EGCG compound from becoming oxidized.

On the other hand, the leaves are fermented to make oolong tea and black tea. The fermentation converts the available EGCG into other chemicals, which are less effective in fighting diseases.

Besides its numerous health benefits, green tea is found to be useful when attempting to lose weight.

There is a lot of evidence supporting the weight loss properties of green tea. One study found that drinking a combination of caffeine and green tea extract burned more calories than drinking only caffeine.

Green Tea Summary

•Green tea has been used to treat everything from headaches, insomnia, and digestive problems. Most recently it's been looked at to help cure cancer.

•Since ancient times the Chinese have used green tea as a traditional medicine in the treatment of a wide range of ailments ranging from depression and insomnia to stomachaches and headaches.

•Studies have consistently shown that Chinese men and women who regularly drank green tea showed a sixty percent lower risk of developing esophageal cancer.

•Additional studies have indicated that green tea is also responsible for lowering the ratio between bad cholesterol (LDL) and good cholesterol (HDL) and also lowering total cholesterol levels in the body.

•Green tea is considered an effective cure for high cholesterol levels, lowered immune system function, cancer, infections, high blood pressure, cardiovascular problems, and rheumatoid arthritis.

•Recent studies have proved that EGCG is two times as powerful as resveratrol, an ingredient in red wine that is known to counter the ill effects of a high-fat diet.

•There is a lot of evidence supporting the weight loss properties of green tea. One study found that drinking a combination of caffeine and green tea extract burned more calories than drinking only caffeine.

BLACK PEPPER

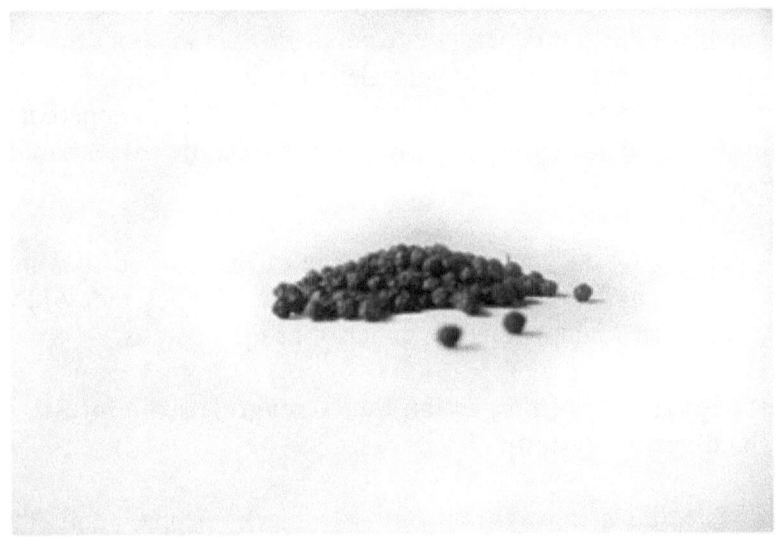

Black Pepper is a popular spice that will stimulate your taste buds and prevent a number of digestive problems.

Reach for the pepper shaker rather than the salt and you'll know it's a bit of health you're shaking onto your plate.

Salt can be very harmful if you have too much, but black pepper on the other hand, is very good for health when used at the table and while cooking.

Black pepper was considered valuable in ancient times and was used as currency.

It was also offered to the gods as a sacrifice.

We are very lucky today to find black pepper in abundance. It is not very expensive and it is not seasonal.

The pepper plant is a huge woody vine that grows higher than 30 feet. It grows in the tropics in humid and hot climates.

Once planted, the plants bear white small flowers in about three to four years. These white flowers develop into berries that are known as peppercorns that are green in color. These peppercorns are further dried and ground to give us the spice that we know as black pepper.

Black pepper not only enhances the taste of the many dishes it is added to, but its benefits go far beyond that. Studies today have proven that black pepper has a number of health benefits.

Black pepper helps in digestion and strengthens the intestines and the digestive system.

Your taste buds are stimulated by black pepper and this stimulation, in turn, helps the stomach increase the secretion of hydrochloric acid, helping to improve the digestion of food once it has reached the stomach.

If the stomach doesn't have enough acids for digestion it leads to indigestion, heartburn and various other problems.

Black pepper helps reduce these problems.

Intestinal gas is also reduced when black pepper is added to your food.

This too is a result of more acid being produced in the stomach.

Black pepper is said to have antibacterial and antioxidant properties that are very vital for fighting diseases.

Black pepper tastes best when ground just before being added to the food and that is one reason why most cooks grind their own peppercorns.

Pepper is easily available at all leading supermarkets, spice boards, organic markets and now even on the Internet.

Fresh peppercorn ground at home enhances the taste of food.

Most folks don't know this but peppercorn skin stimulates your metabolism and helps you maintain a healthier and slimmer body.

The varieties of black pepper are enormous and range from ones that are inexpensive to gourmet black pepper.

You do not have to buy pepper that is very expensive. All you need to do is to buy a brand from a reputable company that sells top quality foods.

Black Pepper Summary

•Black Pepper is a popular spice that will stimulate your taste buds and prevent a number of digestive problems.

•Black pepper helps in digestion and strengthens the intestines and the digestive system.

•Intestinal gas is also reduced when black pepper is added to your food.

•Black pepper is said to have antibacterial and antioxidant properties that are very vital for fighting diseases.

•Most folks don't know this but peppercorn skin stimulates your metabolism and helps you maintain a healthier and slimmer body.

GARLIC

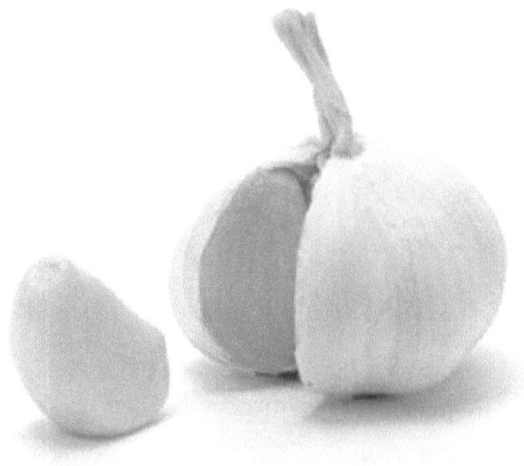

Called the "wonder drug" in the world of natural medicine, and considered to be the first Superfood.

Garlic has been used to treat everything from the common cold to the Bubonic Plague - And It goes great with almost any meal.

Garlic has long been known for its smell, its pungent flavor and its use in many recipes.

It is a favorite with many cultures throughout the world.

For ages, natural health specialists have looked at garlic as a wonder drug.

The general consensus is that the stronger the aroma and flavor, the greater the value garlic has as a medicine..

It is the sulfur compounds in garlic that give it this healing ability and it is the same sulfur that gives it its smell and taste.

Of course, it is not a universal cure for everything, but garlic is something you can consume daily for better overall health.

Buying garlic is easy.

Buy garlic which has the most pungent smell and looks the freshest.

The strong smell is a good indication of the sulfur content of the pod.

Garlic is available in many forms like garlic salt, garlic powder, and garlic paste. You can even make the paste at home and keep it for ready use.

There is an ongoing debate about the quality of organic garlic over the normal kind.

Health enthusiasts feel that the organic variety has more sulfur content and therefore is far superior in healing.

Others would rather not get into an argument and much prefer to have garlic supplements that will give them the benefits of garlic without the problem of garlic breath.

Modern research has found garlic to be useful even as a mosquito repellant as well as having very powerful antibiotic properties.

There is a small downside to all these wonderful benefits of garlic.

Raw garlic is extremely strong and eating too much of this food item can cause problems in a sensitive digestive system.

Then there are those who are allergic to garlic, rare though it is. But in these rare cases garlic can cause skin rashes, fever and, headaches.

Garlic is a natural blood thinner or anticoagulant so it is not advised to have too much in any form, whether supplements, as part of your food, or raw.

This is especially true before surgery of any kind.

For the supplements, ensure that you buy the best brands so you get the best quality and the maximum benefits.

Garlic Summary

•Garlic has been used to treat everything from the common cold to the Bubonic Plague - And It goes great with almost any meal.

•Of course, it is not a universal cure for everything, but garlic is something you can consume daily for better overall health.

•Modern research has found garlic to be useful even as a mosquito repellant as well as having very powerful antibiotic properties.

GINGER

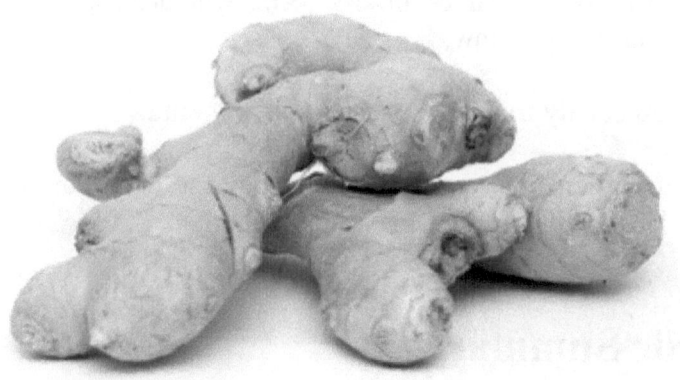

The fragrant, aromatic and pungent ginger root is really a rhizome that grows wild in the moist tropical jungles of India and southeastern Asia from where it has originated.

Today, it is also grown commercially in many subtropical areas.

Ginger has long been used in cooking and medicine, both in India and China. It has been used to remedy a number of ailments for thousands of years.

In Europe, ginger's antiseptic properties and high sulfur content made it a popular antidote for the plague.

Asian cultures have used ginger frequently in medicinal brews and decoctions for a whole range of ailments. It may well be its medicinal properties that helped ginger find its way into so many different foods.

Ginger can be consumed fresh, dried, canned, ground or pickled.

Romans introduced ginger to northern Europe, where it became a popular ingredient in medieval cooking. To this day ginger is used in traditional biscuits, cakes, and sweet dishes.

With ethnic eating influencing eating habits of today's society, ginger's rich, aromatic, pungent, warm flavor in curries and stir fry have made this something found in many households.

Ginger has both stimulating and antiseptic properties which make it increase circulation, relieve colds, coughs, chills and fevers in addition to combating flu.

Studies are even being carried out on ginger's ability to remedy and reduce heart disease.

Traditional medicine has a great many uses for ginger - from healing upset stomachs and diarrhea to nausea, arthritis, and colic.

Villagers in India still use ginger for curing colds and fever, preventing tetanus at childbirth, and nausea during pregnancy.

Many frequent travelers believe that ginger can be prevent motion sickness as well, or better than drugs.

While these claims are being investigated scientifically, chewing a bit of ginger or eating it in a dish before a flight can't hurt anyone.

Ginger and ginger products are available today as extracts, capsules, oils, and tinctures.

Ginger has become so popular that most grocery stores and supermarkets sell it fresh year round. You won't have trouble finding ginger.

Chefs around the world have begun using ginger in imaginative ways in meals and desserts. It is so versatile that it can be used in vegetables, meat, fish or sweet dishes.

It is truly worth using this fragrant, medicinal herb not only for its great taste and aroma but also to improve your health.

Ginger Summary

●Ginger has both stimulating and antiseptic properties which make it increase circulation, relieve colds, coughs, chills and fevers in addition to combating flu.

●Studies are even being carried out on ginger's ability to remedy and reduce heart disease.

●Traditional medicine has a great many uses for ginger - from healing upset stomachs and diarrhea to nausea, arthritis, and colic.

●Many frequent travelers believe that ginger can be prevent motion sickness as well, or better than drugs.

BASIL

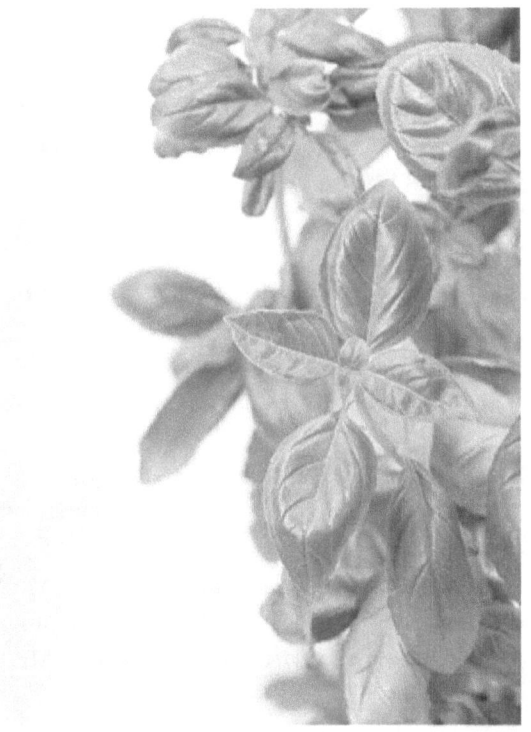

The use of herbs in everyday cooking has become the norm rather than the exception.

Of course herbs add flavor to your food, but they also have therapeutic value.

Basil is one such herb and is characterized by its slightly minty flavor.

This aromatic herb is especially popular with chefs.

Basil is so easy to grow that growing your own is no chore at all.

Fresh basil is also inexpensive if you wish to buy it from the store.

If fresh basil is not available, all you have to do is make a trip to your local supermarket, farmers market, or a store that sells health food where dried basil is sold.

The nutritional value of basil cannot be underestimated.

Basil is rich in vitamins A and C and contains elements like potassium, magnesium, and iron, as also substances like phosphorous and calcium.

The word basil comes from the Greek basilikon meaning 'royal'. Basilikon has its root in basileus, the Greek equivalent for king.

That speaks volumes for the importance given to this herb in the culinary world from ancient times and in varied cultures.

Italians embrace basil as a symbol of love, while in India it is a sign of hospitality.

When basil is included in one's diet, the circulatory system is said to function better. The vitamin A that is present in basil makes for a glowing complexion, glossy hair and, keen eyesight.

Besides all the health benefits you get from adding basil to your diet, it is one of the tastiest of herbs. Its versatility, appreciated by the Europeans, especially the Italians, makes them add it generously to many of their dishes.

Whether you choose fresh basil or the dry variety, go for the best and add it generously to your cuisine. This appetizing herb enhances the flavor of your cooking and is good for you. What more could one ask for!

Basil Summary

•Basil is rich in vitamins A and C and contains elements like potassium, magnesium, and iron, as also substances like phosphorous and calcium.

•When basil is included in one's diet, the circulatory system is said to function better. The vitamin A that is present in basil makes for a glowing complexion, glossy hair and, keen eyesight.

CINNAMON

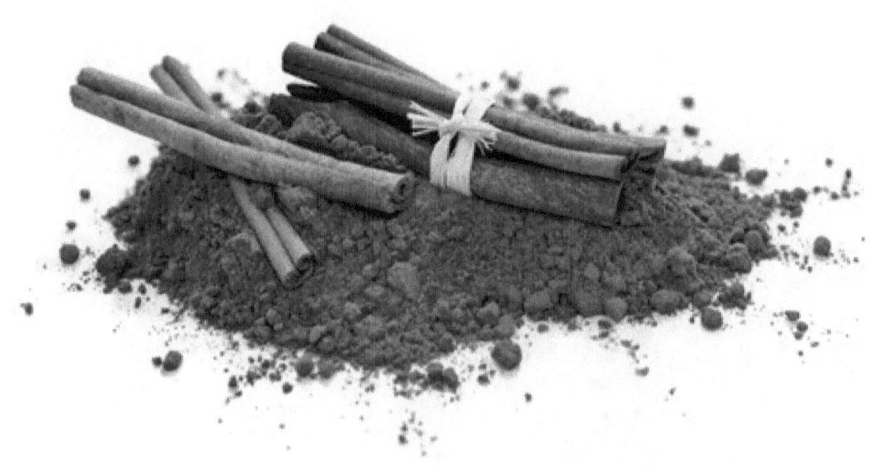

For over four thousand years, ancient Chinese, Indians and Egyptians have used cinnamon as a medicine for various ailments and in cooking.

It is not clear whether it was used in cooking first or as a medicine first.

Whatever its origins, this wonderful aromatic spice is known for being antiseptic, anti-inflammatory, astringent, and healing. It has been traditionally used for gastrointestinal ailments, heart problems, diabetes and, a myriad other ailments.

The Egyptians even used cinnamon for embalming.

Cinnamon spice is the aromatic bark of the Cinnamomum verum tree, belonging to the laurel family and native to Sri Lanka.

Other trees from the same families and aromatic cassia are found in China and southern Asia. Due to its demand, cinnamon today is commercially grown in many tropical countries.

Arabs introduced the fragrant spice to the Europeans using the famous overland spice route. It has been fought over, traded for, used as currency and at times it has been more expensive than gold.

Today it is cheap and easily available as curled dried bark called quills or powdered and you can pick them up in grocery stores everywhere.

Ancient and modern cultures have used and continue to use cinnamon for its wonderful aroma and taste in cooking and its great medicinal properties.

It has traditionally been used for gastrointestinal disorders, flatulence, morning sickness, diabetes, heart problems, high blood pressure and its anti-inflammatory, antiseptic, astringent and food preserving properties.

Scientific studies have confirmed the many beneficial effects of this spice. The properties have been attributed to the basic aromatic oils, cinnamaldehyde, cinnamyl acetate, cinnamyl alcohol and other volatile substances found in the bark.

A recent study published in the Journal of Diabetes Care found that 1/2 a teaspoon of Cinnamon significantly lowered blood sugar levels in diabetics.

Science has also confirmed that cinnamon helps reduce cholesterol and blood pressure, and various other beneficial effects.

Let's take a look at some of them.

It acts as a digestive aid as it is antiflatulent, antibacterial, antifungal and antiseptic.

All of this aids digestion and prevents infection and discomfort.

Cinnamon also relieves aches and pains like menstrual cramping, muscle and, joint pains and stiffness.

It improves circulation by stimulating the brain and prevents platelets from clotting unnecessarily.

Cinnamon also reduces cholesterol in the blood and regulates blood pressure.

It gives relief from colds, congestion, and allergies.

It relieves arthritic and rheumatic pain due to its anti-inflammatory properties.

Being antibacterial, it prevents urinary tract infections, gum disease, and tooth decay.

Cinnamon alleviates liver complications and helps bile absorption.

With so many beneficial properties and a delightful taste, cinnamon should be made a regular part of your diet.

Cinnamon Summary

●Cinnamon is known for being antiseptic, anti-inflammatory, astringent, and healing. It has been traditionally used for gastrointestinal ailments, heart problems, diabetes and, a myriad other ailments.

●A recent study published in the Journal of Diabetes Care found that 1/2 a teaspoon of Cinnamon significantly lowered blood sugar levels in diabetics.

●Science has also confirmed that cinnamon helps reduce cholesterol and blood pressure, and various other beneficial effects.

●Cinnamon acts as a digestive aid as it is antiflatulent, antibacterial, antifungal and antiseptic.

●Cinnamon also relieves aches and pains like menstrual cramping, muscle and, joint pains and stiffness.

●Cinnamon improves circulation by stimulating the brain and prevents platelets from clotting unnecessarily.

●Cinnamon also reduces cholesterol in the blood and regulates blood pressure.

●Cinnamon gives relief from colds, congestion, and allergies.

●Cinnamon relieves arthritic and rheumatic pain due to its anti-inflammatory properties.

●Being antibacterial, Cinnamon prevents urinary tract infections, gum disease, and tooth decay.

●Cinnamon alleviates liver complications and helps bile absorption.

BILBERRY

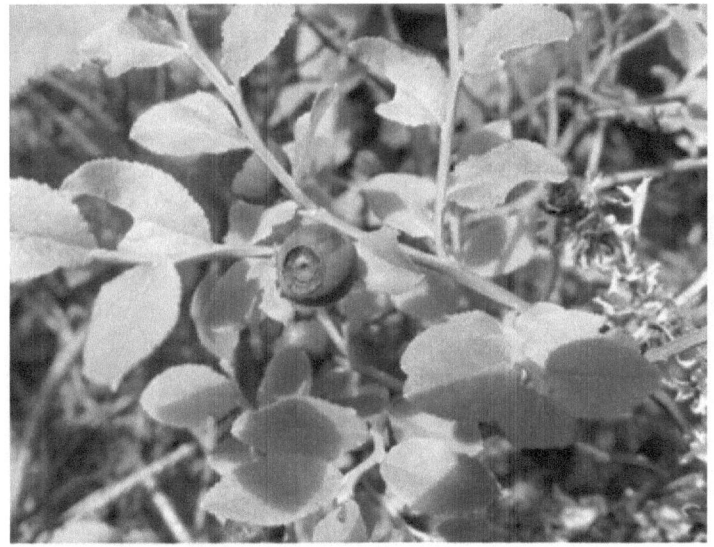

Keen eyesight will be yours with this sweet berry.

Those who regularly indulge in the bilberry can also expect to noticed a reduction in varicose veins.

The bilberry, native to Europe and North America, is a close relative of the blueberry and bears the botanical name actinium myrtillus.

The sweet, blue, or blackish fruit grows on bushes that best thrive in soils that are both acidic and damp. From ancient times, the bilberry has been known for its medicinal properties. Apart from the berries, the leaves too are used in the healing process.

Perhaps the most remarkable feature of the bilberry is that it is said to sharpen vision at night.

World War II pilots found that the more bilberries they consumed, the keener was their vision while flying sorties at night.

Scientific research has proven that consumption of bilberries does not merely slow declining vision, but actually results in keener eyesight.

As early as the sixteenth century, honey was added to bilberries to form a syrup. This syrup called rob was administered to those suffering from diarrhea.

Our ancestors seemed to have used the bilberry as an antidote for a number of medical problems including diabetes and indigestion. Today the effect of the berry on vision is what is being most researched.

Researchers hold that the phytochemicals in the bilberry are responsible not only for lowering of the blood pressure but also for helping in the prevention of clot formation.

According to studies, the nervous system reaps benefits too.

Bilberries also help improve blood flow and overall circulatory system health.

Scientists claim that the antioxidants in bilberry are fifty times more effective than Vitamin E and ten times more efficacious than Vitamin C.

Eating bilberries help improve the efficiency of the vascular system, enabling the connected organs to function better.

For instance, the circulatory system shows an increase in blood circulation. As a result, your organs perform more efficiently and visual acuteness is enhanced.

In places where fresh bilberries are scarce, you can use bilberry supplements.

However, it is best to get your hands on fresh bilberries if you can.

Including bilberries in your daily diet will do wonders for your health.

If it is clarity of vision that you want and the efficient functioning of the nervous and cardiovascular systems, don't pass on bilberries!

Bilberry Summary

•Those who regularly indulge in the bilberry can also expect to noticed a reduction in varicose veins

•Scientific research has proven that consumption of bilberries does not merely slow declining vision, but actually results in keener eyesight.

•Researchers hold that the phytochemicals in the bilberry are responsible not only for lowering of the blood pressure but also for helping in the prevention of clot formation.

•Bilberries also help improve blood flow and overall circulatory system health.

MILK THISTLE

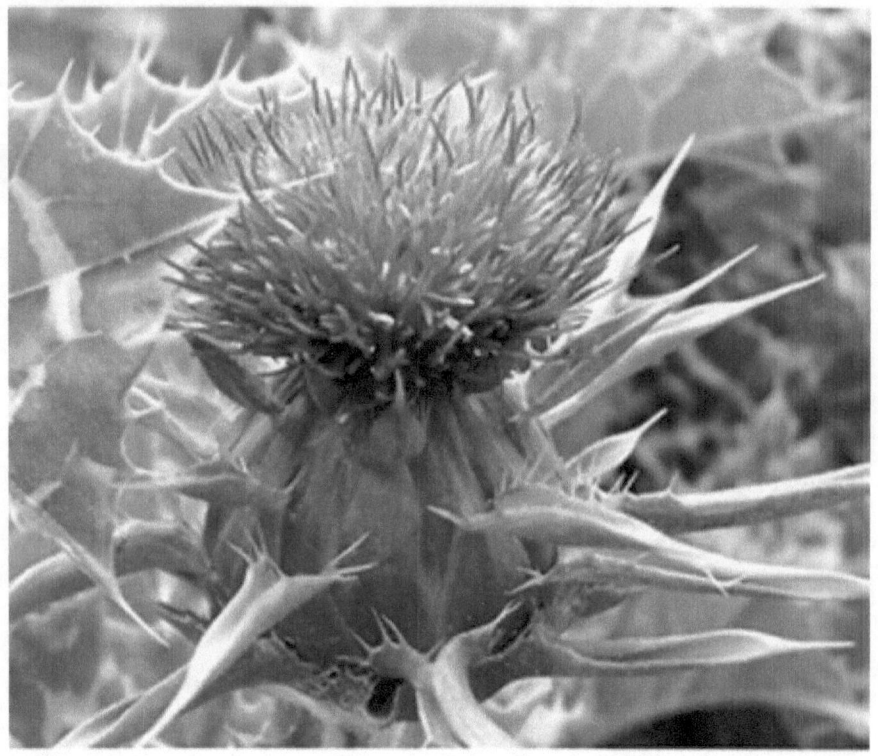

Milk thistle is a member of the sunflower family, and it's used to remove toxins from the liver.

It's so powerful that it's even used as an antidote for poisonous mushrooms.

Milk thistle, also known as Mary thistle and holy thistle, is a prickly plant, native to the Mediterranean region but now growing in the wild all over the world.

In the ancient world, it was a must on every healer's shelf.

Milk thistle has been used for thousands of years as a tonic, purifier, and cure for various disorders especially liver ailments.

Its scientific name is Silybum Marianum from where its active ingredients, silymarin and silibinin found in concentrated amounts in the black fruit, get their name.

Research and studies have confirmed these ancient healers' claims.

They have found that the active ingredient, silymarin, helps protect the liver from damage, improve its function and reverse and heal damaged livers due to cirrhosis or hepatitis.

It has also shown to improve the gallbladder function.

Strong indications show Milk thistle can lower cholesterol, fight cancer, heal digestive disorders, relieve allergies, and help the absorption of insulin in diabetic patients with liver damage.

Milk thistle also has very high antioxidant properties.

Milk thistle is such a powerful healer that an injectable form is used to help people who've ingested poisonous mushrooms.

This is due to its ability to rapidly eliminate toxins from the body and its ability to protect and heal the liver and gallbladder and influence bile secretion.

Milk thistle is also being studied as a therapy for liver damage caused by chemotherapy.

Milk Thistle should be used as a concentrated extract.

Milk thistle teas are very low in silymarin and silibinin, and these substances are not water soluble and will not have the desired effect.

Moreover, all parts except the seeds have negligible amounts of silymarins.

Milk thistle appear at the end of summer and due to the properties of the active ingredients cannot be processed at home. Treatments usually require 400 to 600 milligrams a day to be taken in three equal doses.

A lot of research on Milk thistle is being carried out on various fronts.

These include the effects of the milk thistle in chronic hepatitis C, non-alcoholic liver disease, cancer prevention and the treatment of complications in AIDS patients in addition to its liver protecting and poison eliminating properties.

Milk thistle products must be bought from reliable sources and your physician must know about its use, in case of other medication being prescribed.

Milk thistle products are available in most natural and health food stores in addition to the Internet providers.

Today it is available as standardized extracts in capsules.

A few side effects have been reported such as mild gastrointestinal disorders, bloating and mild allergies in those allergic to certain plants.

Milk Thistle Summary

●Milk Thistle is so powerful that it's even used as an antidote for poisonous mushrooms.

• The active ingredient in Milk Thistle, silymarin, helps protect the liver from damage, improve its function and reverse and heal damaged livers due to cirrhosis or hepatitis.

• Milk Thistle has shown to improve the gallbladder function.

• Strong indications show Milk thistle can lower cholesterol, fight cancer, heal digestive disorders, relieve allergies, and help the absorption of insulin in diabetic patients with liver damage.

ECHINACEA

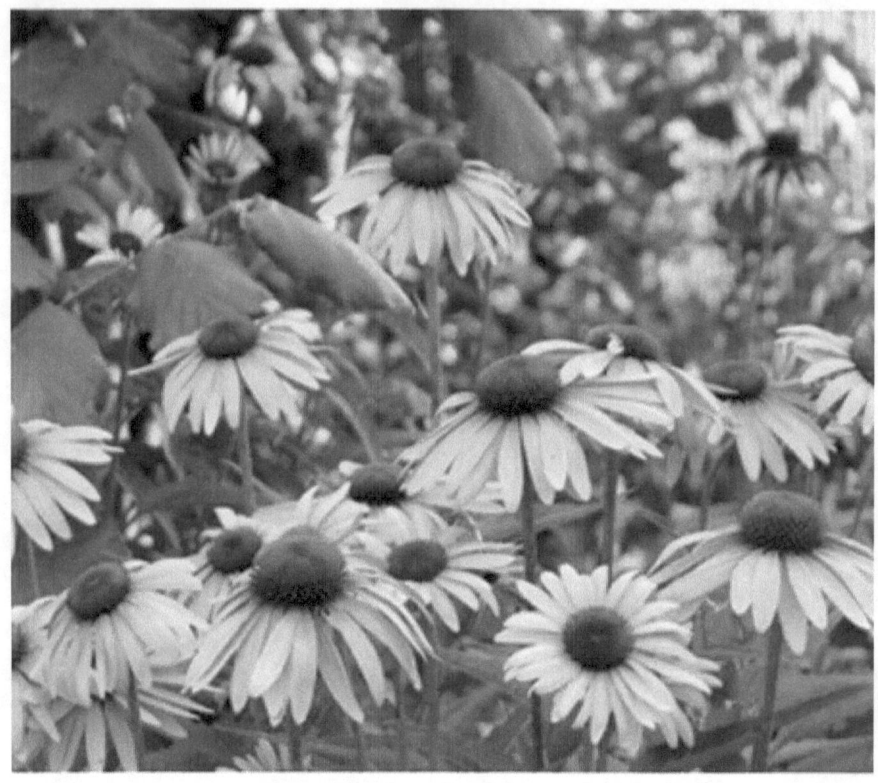

Tired of getting laid up with a cold every year? Take Echinacea to boost your immune system.

Echinacea is part of the plethora of herbs and natural remedies that are available on the market today.

Echinacea is one of the better-known herbs, and it lives up to its reputation as being a cold, flu and common infection fighter.

Echinacea is a purple cone-shaped flower and can be found in nine varieties or species. There are three types used for medicinal purposes: Echinacea purpurea, Echinacea angustifolia, and Echinacea pallida.

Echinacea is available in many forms - pills, capsules, tablets, liquids, gels, and tincture. You can brew it as tea in its dried form. Then there is the cream variant which is good for sunburns and skin problems.

Echinacea is used for many products and preparations and every part of the plant is used - the leaves, stems, and roots and of course the flower itself.

There are specific types of Echinacea used for fighting bacteria, stimulating the immune system, and fighting various strains of viruses that invade our body from time to time.

Every day there are little mishaps just waiting to happen. These can be anything from minor burns to canker sores, boils, eczema, abscesses, cuts, scrapes, and other related skin afflictions. Echinacea is very effective when applied directly to these problems or taken orally to boost the repair and healing of the wound.

One of the most difficult problems to diagnose has been chronic fatigue syndrome and Echinacea has shown to help with that.

Interferon is a substance known to fight viruses in our body. Echinacea is considered to be effective in giving the cells that produce this interferon a boost so that they are able to do their job efficiently.

The use of Echinacea is very helpful in reducing the incidence of colds and flu in our body. it works best if taken at the very first symptoms so you can knock it out early.

If you already have a cold then Echinacea will bring down the severity and the duration.

Common respiratory problems like a strep throat, sinusitis, and even bronchitis can also be helped by taking Echinacea.

You need to know exactly what health problem you're trying to address when shopping for Echinacea. Different Echinacea products are formulated to relieve differed health issues so make sure you read the label before buying an Echinacea product.

Echinacea Summary

•Echinacea is one of the better-known herbs, and it lives up to its reputation as being a cold, flu and common infection fighter.

•There are specific types of Echinacea used for fighting bacteria, stimulating the immune system, and fighting various strains of viruses that invade our body from time to time.

•One of the most difficult problems to diagnose has been chronic fatigue syndrome and Echinacea has shown to help with that.

•Interferon is a substance known to fight viruses in our body. Echinacea is considered to be effective in giving the cells that produce this interferon a boost so that they are able to do their job efficiently.

•Common respiratory problems like a strep throat, sinusitis, and even bronchitis can also be helped by taking Echinacea.

ST. JOHN'S WORT

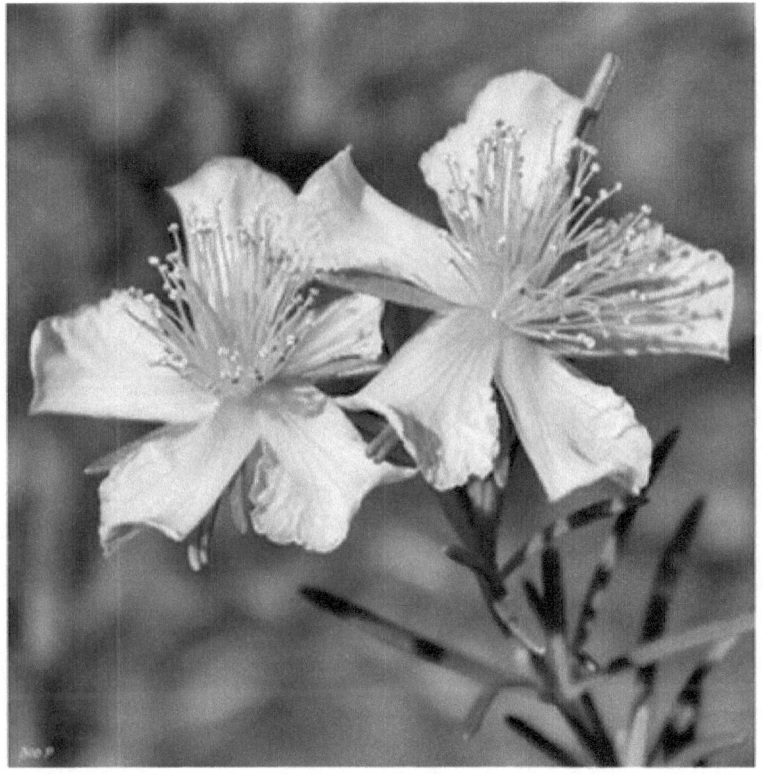

Depression is becoming a major problem in many countries.

What's unfortunate is the fact that so many people just do not want to seek treatment for it.

Diseases of the mind still have a stigma attached to them. Many people feel weak for seeking treatment for them.

What is fortunate, however, is the growing awareness of alternative therapies and medicines to treat depression.

St. John's Wort is one herb that has proved very beneficial in this area.

The best part is that St. John's Wort treats both depression and anxiety without the need for prescription drugs which come with their own side effects.

St. John's Wort is a great mood elevator and so many who have taken it are thrilled with the results.

The botanical name for St. John's Wort is Hypericum perforatum, but the common name it's known by comes from St. John the Baptist.

St. John was born in June and it is in this month that the plant starts to flower with golden blooms.

The meaning of 'wort' is plant, so effectively, it means St. John's plant.

It is a perennial plant and keeps growing back every year from just one single plant. In fact, it's almost a weed, growing wild all over Europe where it has had a field day for thousands of years.

St. John's Wort has a long history as a medicinal plant.

In fact, the father of medicine, Hippocrates is said to have used the herb for conditions like jaundice, dysentery, TB, insomnia, colds, and hemorrhage.

Recently, medical science has discovered a compound in St. John's Wort called hypericin. This compound works on the brain and causes a calm, soothing effect.

In fact, it works very much like an antidepressant, without the dangers associated with taking strong medication like that.

Very often, this herb is the only medication you need if your depression is mild or moderate.

St. John's Wort also increases circulation and helps you sleep better.

You can get St. John's Wort as capsules and tea and it is available in a range of strengths.

You can buy it over the counter in most stores.

The standardized dose is 300 mg which has a hypericin concentration of 0.3.

You could also drink St. John's Wort as a tea. Pour hot water over 2 teaspoons of the dried herb and steep for around 10 minutes, strain and drink mixed with sugar or honey.

You can also make a massage oil by steeping the St. John's Wort in olive oil and using it to relieve arthritic pain and inflammation. It is also effective for sprains and bruises.

St. John's Wort Summary

●St. John's Wort treats both depression and anxiety without the need for prescription drugs which come with their own side effects.

●Recently, medical science has discovered a compound in St. John's Wort called hypericin. This compound works on the brain and causes a calm, soothing effect.

●St. John's Wort increases circulation and helps you sleep better.

●You can also make a massage oil by steeping the St. John's Wort in olive oil and using it to relieve arthritic pain and inflammation. It is also effective for sprains and bruises.

66

GINKGO BILOBA

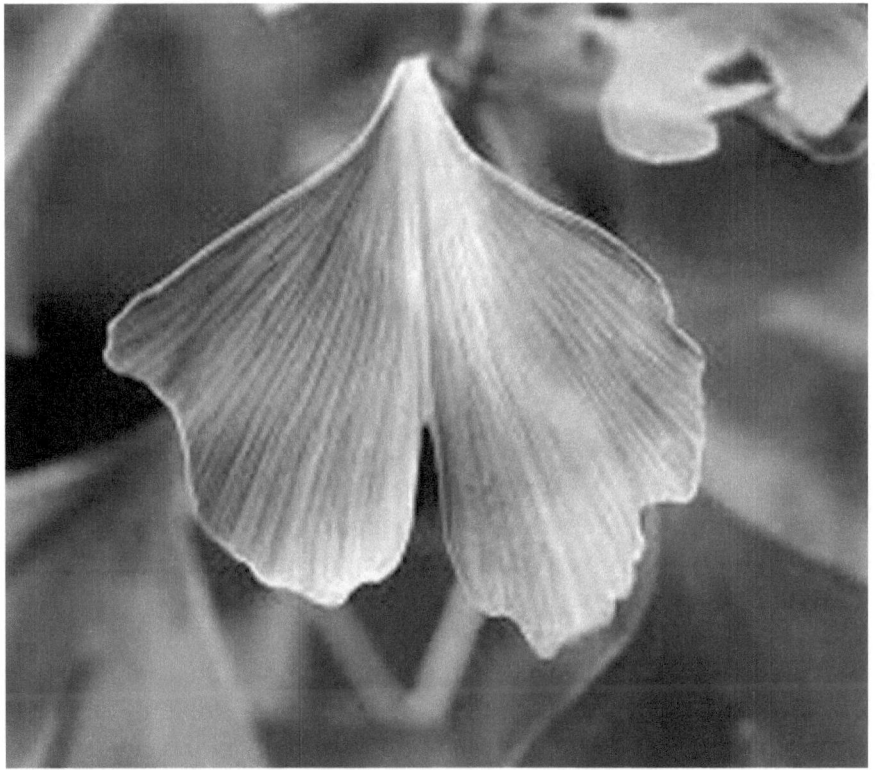

For 1000's of years people have been using Ginkgo Biloba to improve blood flow, increase sexual energy, improve longevity, boost memory, and get rid of depression

Ginkgo Biloba has emerged from being an ornamental tree in manicured gardens to a modern-day Superfood for your brain.

The Ginkgo tree, also known as the maidenhair tree, is gorgeous and ornamental with its fan-shaped dark green leaves which turn into a golden, deep yellow in autumn, leaving the beautiful, patterned, silver branches leafless in winter.

It has a long life and is said to be able to live a thousand years and geologically has been in existence for a hundred and fifty million years.

It has miraculously survived all kinds of natural catastrophes. It is native to southern China, Korea, and Japan.

The Chinese have used both Ginkgo leaves and seeds for centuries to treat all sorts of ailments from circulatory problems to memory enhancement.

The Ginkgo leaf is very well researched. The most commonly used ginkgo product is the concentrated Ginkgo Biloba Extract or GBE which has been standardized.

Research has shown GBE to have both flavonoids and terpenoids, both of which have very strong antioxidant properties which neutralize dangerous free radicals in the human body. Free radicals are responsible for aging, cell destruction and DNA alteration like cancer cells.

Studies have shown that GBE helps blood flow, thus improving circulation. This, in turn, is effective in treating problems arising from decreased blood flow to the brain, especially in the elderly.

With better circulation to the brain, the memory gets better and memory loss is slowed or even improved.

The free radical neutralizing power of Ginkgo aids in the treatment of heart disease, cancer, dementia, and Alzheimer's disease.

That's just the beginning of what Ginkgo can do for you...

Ginkgo use has proven effective in eliminating psoriasis and other skin problems, reversing asthma symptoms, and reducing tinnitus or ringing in the ears.

GBE has also been shown to reduce depression and improving social behavior.

Thinking, memory, and learning have all been improved with regular GBE use.

Retinal damage and age-related macular degeneration due to atherosclerosis have been lessened or halted.

Today herbalists are recommending GBE for anxiety, tension, mood boosting, energizing, vertigo, headaches, high blood pressure and even for erectile dysfunction amongst others.

On a cautionary note, it is important to make sure that the GBE has been properly processed to remove the harmful ginkgolic acid to less than 5 parts per million.

A wide variety of herbalists, pharmacies, nature cure stores in addition to the Internet sell reliable GBE products.

Europe is the largest user of GBE which is sold as the standardized GBE containing 24% flavonoids and 6% terpenoids with less than 5 parts per million of ginkgolic acid. These are available in tinctures, capsules, and tablets.

A few cases of mild adverse reactions to Ginkgo have been reported including mild dizziness, stomach upsets, headaches, and mild skin rash.

Your physician must be told of GBE use so that there is no adverse reaction with other medication especially with blood thinning agents.

Because of its blood thinning properties, GBE use must be discontinued before surgery.

Ginkgo Biloba Summary

●Research has shown Ginkgo Biloba Extract to have both flavonoids and terpenoids, both of which have very strong antioxidant properties which neutralize dangerous free radicals in the human body. Free radicals are responsible for aging, cell destruction and DNA alteration like cancer cells.

●The free radical neutralizing power of Ginkgo aids in the treatment of heart disease, cancer, dementia, and Alzheimer's disease.

●Ginkgo use has proven effective in eliminating psoriasis and other skin problems, reversing asthma symptoms, and reducing tinnitus or ringing in the ears.

●Ginkgo Biloba Extract has also been shown to reduce depression and improving social behavior.

●Thinking, memory, and learning have all been improved with regular Ginkgo Biloba Extract use.

●Retinal damage and age-related macular degeneration due to atherosclerosis have been lessened or halted with Ginkgo Biloba Extract use.

●Herbalists are recommending Ginkgo Biloba Extract for anxiety, tension, mood boosting, energizing, vertigo, headaches, high blood pressure and even for erectile dysfunction amongst others.

BOSWELLIA

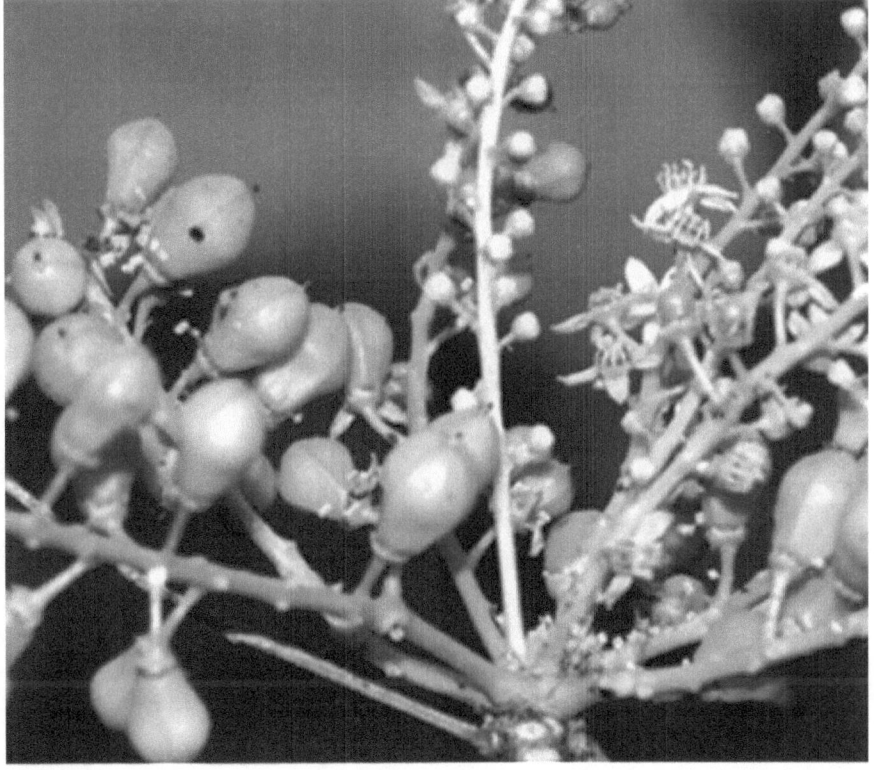

It is called the Indian frankincense and grows wild in the hills in India.

Boswellia is a gummy resin that comes from the bark of the Boswellia Serrata tree and has long been used by Indian medicine men.

Boswellia has found its way into modern medicine and is used to fight inflammation and a whole host of diseases.

Today, the resin is purified and sold in the form of creams or pills.

Unlike NSAID or non-steroidal anti-inflammatory drugs that tend to cause irritation in the stomach, Boswellia provides you with gentle relief.

Boswellia is also very effective for intestine disorders as well as backaches.

How does boswellic acids fight inflammation so well?

Research has found that boswellic acids in Boswellia are responsible for making Boswellia such a great anti-inflammatory substance.

Boswellia has been tested and studies indicate that the reduction in inflammation is because these acids improve the flow of blood to the joints and do not allow the white blood cells to get inflamed.

They also tend to block any kind of chemical reaction that could bring on inflammation.

Thanks to its anti-inflammatory characteristics, Boswellia is a simple, natural remedy you can take for arthritis, back aches, and other joint pain.

When taken orally, Boswellia has been found to relieve ulcerative colitis and Crohn's disease.

Unlike traditional pain relievers, Boswellia is not addictive.

Boswellia can be bought as topical creams, capsules, and tablets.

For pain, the topical cream is very effective. For serious pain or arthritis, this can be complemented with oral doses of the herb.

In the rare case of a rash or nausea, it would be advisable to stop taking Boswellia.

The Boswellia you buy should have a 60% concentration of the herb as this is the standardized level.

Boswellia Summary

●Boswellia has found its way into modern medicine and is used to fight inflammation and a whole host of diseases.

●Boswellia is also very effective for intestine disorders as well as backaches.

●Thanks to its anti-inflammatory characteristics, Boswellia is a simple, natural remedy you can take for arthritis, back aches, and other joint pain.

●When taken orally, Boswellia has been found to relieve ulcerative colitis and Crohn's disease.

BLACK COHOSH

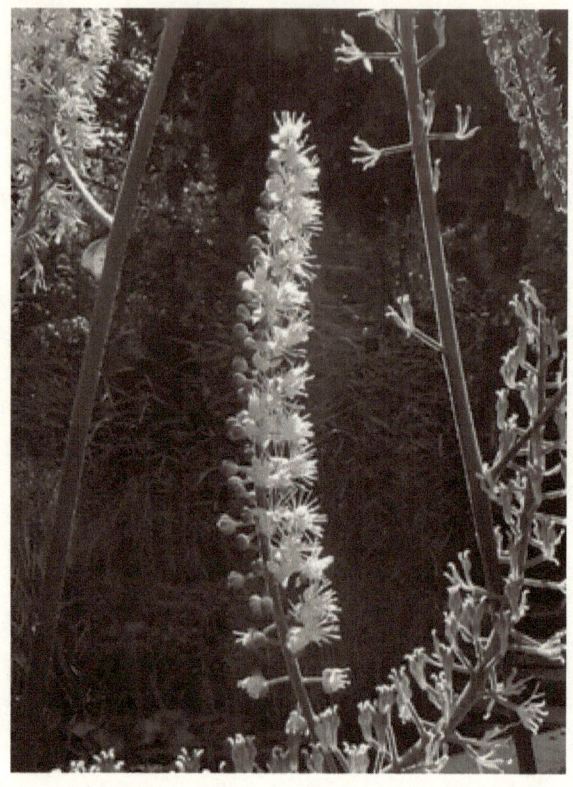

Many women today put their faith in a little plant called black cohosh to help ease female-related problems like menopause and PMS.

This practice that goes back generations.

Way back in the early 1900s, the wildflower called black cohosh was one of the main ingredients used in a famous tonic that helped in curing a large number of female problems.

Black cohosh comes from the buttercup family. It not only helps in menopause and PMS related problems but also helps cure insect bites and eczema.

For many years black cohosh was somewhat forgotten, but today it has become a very popular root again and it is used in herbal treatments to cure hot flashes which are one of the most common symptoms of menopause.

Doctors recommend black cohosh to their patients for the treatment of menopause symptoms when it started becoming apparent that hormone replacement therapy carried a lot of health risks.

Black cohosh can also treat coughs and congestion and it's anti-inflammatory. Plus it's a mild sedative and helps relieve muscle aches.

You can also treat muscle pains and aches using a warm compress, which has been dipped in tea made out of black cohosh.

Black cohosh is able to treat menstrual cramps because of its antispasmodic properties that are effective in easing cramps. It increases the flow of blood to the uterus and reduces the awful, cramping pain.

40 mg of black cohosh should be taken twice a day for PMS symptoms.

This regime should be followed for eight to ten days before your period.

Black cohosh is available in numerous forms that include: capsules, tinctures, dried herbs and tablets. Dried black cohosh herbs are used in the preparation of soothing teas.

When shopping for black cohosh supplements make sure they contain 2.5% triterpene glycosides because that's the active part of the root.

If you are buying black cohosh in liquid form, make sure the product contain 5% triterpene glycosides.

For many, capsules made from freeze-dried black cohosh are the best choice because they tend to be the highest quality.

Black Cohosh Summary

●Black cohosh comes from the buttercup family. It not only helps in menopause and PMS related problems but also helps cure insect bites and eczema.

●Black cohosh can also treat coughs and congestion and it's anti-inflammatory. Plus it's a mild sedative and helps relieve muscle aches.

BEANS

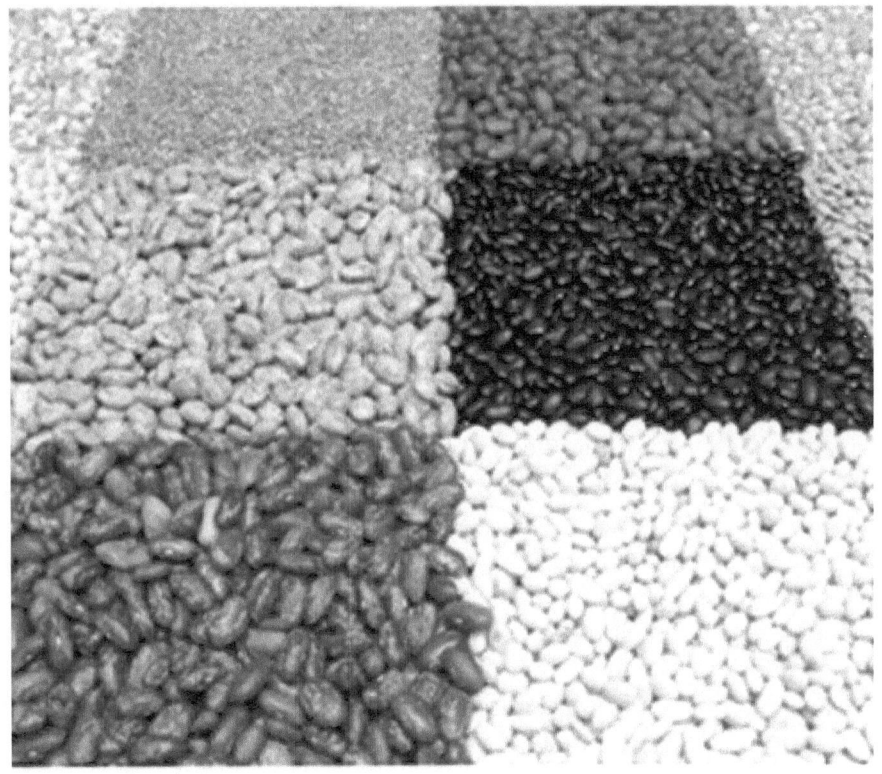

Beans have been a food staple of civilizations for thousands of years.

Every culture has special bean dishes. Whether they are called dal, porotos or just beans, this legume is power packed with nutrition and healing ability.

Beans are so highly regarded in some cultures that they are considered the perfect food.

Beans are packed with vitamins and proteins, are nutritious and fiber-rich.

Beans are also low in calories and fats.

Many vegetarians get most of their proteins from the humble bean!

Research has shown that consuming three to four servings of beans a week or just half a cup a day can help with weight loss, reduce the risk of breast and other cancers, diabetes, and heart disease.

The isoflavones present in the beans are responsible for this.

The high fiber content of beans, both soluble and insoluble, help digestion and elimination.

Beans are also so filling that smaller amounts are required to reach the 'satisfaction level'.

Beans are not only cheap but versatile to cook with. The varieties of beans available on the market make them a must on every kitchen shelf whether dried, canned or frozen.

When canning and refrigeration were not available the humble dried bean could be stored for years.

The wonderful properties of beans are being studied by nutritionists and scientists all over the world and some amazing facts have come to light.

Beans have much of the goodness of meat and milk without any cholesterol.

Beans are a rich source of potassium and are low in sodium, thus helping to ward off high blood pressure and strokes.

The high protein content of beans provides good nourishment for muscle, bone and tissue development.

The complex carbohydrates in beans satisfy hunger for longer periods and provide long-lasting energy. The antioxidants help against aging while healing and fighting disease.

Fiber in beans provides roughage to absorb and eliminate toxins and waste products from the body.

The soluble fiber in beans trap fats and cholesterol and helps eliminate them, protecting the heart and other organs. Beans also help keep your bowel movements regular which lowers your risk of getting colon cancer.

Beans are loaded with Vitamin B9 or folate. This B family vitamin is essential for pregnant women and the developing baby. Folates are known to be cardiovascular protectors and reduce tumors and the formation of cancer cells.

There is some indication that the folate in beans can help reverse lungs damaged due to smoking.

With all these benefits why not eat beans every day to keep the doctor away!

Beans Summary

•Research has shown that consuming three to four servings of beans a week or just half a cup a day can help with weight loss, reduce the risk of breast and other cancers, diabetes, and heart disease.

•The high fiber content of beans, both soluble and insoluble, help digestion and elimination.

●Beans have much of the goodness of meat and milk without any cholesterol.

●Beans are a rich source of potassium and are low in sodium, thus helping to ward off high blood pressure and strokes.

●The high protein content of beans provides good nourishment for muscle, bone and tissue development.

●The complex carbohydrates in beans satisfy hunger for longer periods and provide long-lasting energy. The antioxidants help against aging while healing and fighting disease.

●The soluble fiber in beans trap fats and cholesterol and helps eliminate them, protecting the heart and other organs. Beans also help keep your bowel movements regular which lowers your risk of getting colon cancer.

●Beans are loaded with Vitamin B9 or folate. This B family vitamin is essential for pregnant women and the developing baby. Folates are known to be cardiovascular protectors and reduce tumors and the formation of cancer cells.

BLUEBERRIES

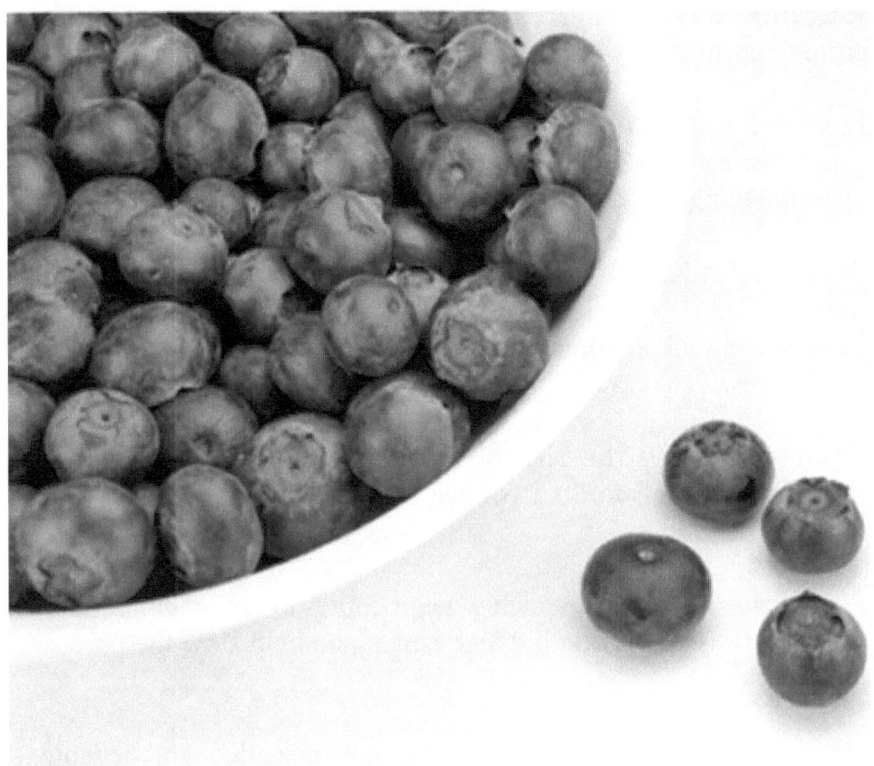

Making your plate a rainbow-colored spread, should be the new health mantra.

You should be eating at least five servings of vegetables and fruits a day and most nutrition experts agree that this should consist of a variety of colors.

If you are looking for fruits packed with a lot of goodness, think blue.

Blueberries are said to be good cancer-fighting agents as they contain a large number of antioxidants which are pivotal in the war against cancer in the body.

Blueberries are also proving to be very good for the mind.

Research has discovered that Blueberries have memory-enhancing qualities and are said to protect the brain.

Blueberries are full of phytochemicals called phenolics and anthocyanins on which studies are being conducted to determine their antiaging and their anticancer properties.

Blueberries also help ensure your urinary tract works well.

Let's take a look at some other health benefits you can enjoy from blueberries....

Besides reducing the risk of heart diseases, Blueberries also improve eyesight, build stronger and better blood vessels, and help your memory.

Blueberries also pack a punch when it comes to antioxidants. They are great to fight off and prevent cancer and help slow the process of aging.

An important antioxidant in blueberries is called anthocyanin. You'll find this antioxidant in blackberries, apples, grapes, red cabbage and radishes as well.

But blueberries can beat the whole lot hands down when it comes to the amounts of anthocyanin they contain.

Blueberries can also help you see in the dark - it makes night vision better and strengthens the blood vessels behind the eye which makes macular degeneration slow down.

What's more, they are a weight watchers delight as they are low in calories.

You could have a whole cup and it would be just 80 calories. Plus, you'll get a number of vitamins as well as iron and potassium.

There's more.

Blueberries give you dietary fiber as well. You'll get a full 4 grams of fiber in every serving of blueberries. That's a whole lot of goodness to pack into one bowl!

Blueberries Summary

●Research has discovered that Blueberries have memory-enhancing qualities and are said to protect the brain.

●Blueberries also help ensure your urinary tract works well.

●Besides reducing the risk of heart diseases, Blueberries also improve eyesight, build stronger and better blood vessels, and help your memory.

●Blueberries can also help you see in the dark - it makes night vision better and strengthens the blood vessels behind the eye which makes macular degeneration slow down.

CRANBERRY

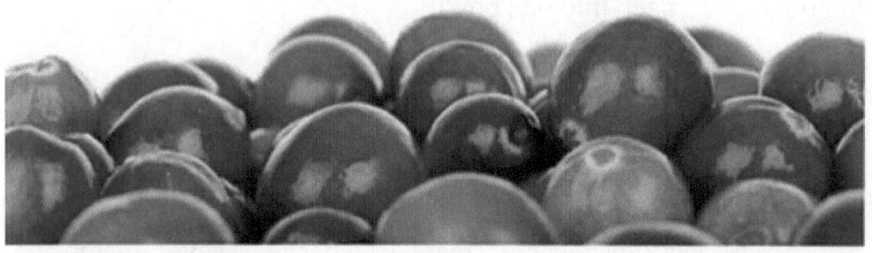

The cranberry, also known as American cranberry and bog cranberry is native to North America and grows in the wild.

Today it is being widely cultivated. The fruits ripen in autumn to a beautiful deep red.

No Thanksgiving meal is complete without one or more cranberry dishes.

Historically, this red berry was used by the local Native Americans and later the European settlers as a medicinal herb and for making juices, drinks, and wines.

Cranberry fruit and leaves were used as teas and decoctions to heal wounds, soothe gastrointestinal disorders, cure diabetes and alleviate liver complaints.

Modern research has indeed shown the cranberry to be beneficial to your health in various ways.

Cranberries have been found to contain very high doses of beneficial antioxidants which neutralize and destroy the

harmful free radicals responsible for aging and disease within the body.

Your body naturally produces antioxidants but it's typically not sufficient most of the time due to disease or stress and other factors.

Experts and nutritionists all agree that a diet rich in fruits and vegetables is beneficial for your health. Fruits like the cranberry are so packed with nutrients and antioxidants that they've earned a reputation as a Superfood that you should be eating more of.

Cranberries provide a variety of nutrients that increase vitality, fitness and, health while helping to ward off certain ailments like urinary tract infections, stomach ulcers caused by certain bacteria, E. coli infections, and gum disease.

Cranberries even have anti-carcinogenic properties. All these properties are due to the proanthocyanidins or PACs present in cranberries which prevent the bacteria from sticking to the walls of the digestive tract.

The antioxidant, vitamin-packed cranberry is seriously being studied by researchers and laboratories for its various beneficial properties.

The NCCAM and National Institute of Diabetes and Digestive and Kidney Disease has been researching the cranberry as a way to prevent urinary tract infection and have found promising data.

The National Institute for Dental and Craniofacial Research is also studying the properties of the cranberry to prevent dental plaque. So a cranberry miracle toothpaste or mouthwash may happen in the future!

Cranberries are available year-round, fresh, frozen, canned or as pure juices and mixed juices.

A glass of Cranberry juice or a small bowl full of berries a day could help you achieve health, vitality, beauty and keep disease at bay.

For those who like it in dishes, there's Cranberry sauce, pudding, and topping for other desserts. Of course, those who prefer supplements can find it as teas, extracts, tablets, and capsules from health shops.

Cranberry Summary

●Cranberries have been found to contain very high doses of beneficial antioxidants which neutralize and destroy the harmful free radicals responsible for aging and disease within the body.

●Cranberries provide a variety of nutrients that increase vitality, fitness and, health while helping to ward off certain ailments like urinary tract infections, stomach ulcers caused by certain bacteria, E. coli infections, and gum disease.

●Cranberries even have anti-carcinogenic properties. All these properties are due to the proanthocyanidins or PACs present in cranberries which prevent the bacteria from sticking to the walls of the digestive tract.

DONG QUAI

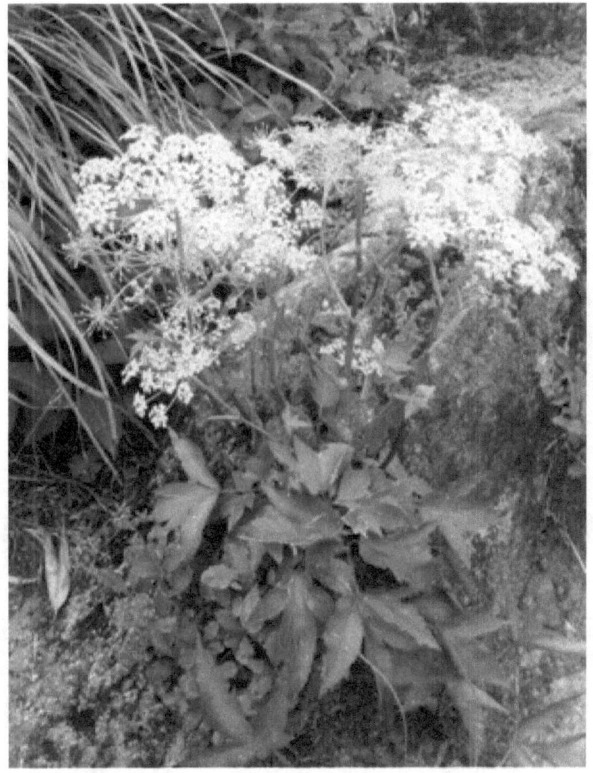

This remedy is as old as the hills and has been used by Asian women for thousands of years as a tonic for the reproductive system.

Dong Quai is a herb that has been regularly used in countries like China and Japan and probably ranks just below ginseng when it comes to the extent of its usage.

What is dong quai?

In Japan, it comes from the Angelica acutiloba plant's root and in China, it is obtained from the root of the angelica sinensis. Both these plants have stems that are hollow and grow up to a height of eight feet and have white flowers that bloom in clusters in the shape of an umbrella.

The flowers of both these species resemble Queen Anne's lace.

Dong Quai is used more among women as it helps improve uterine health, which in turn regularizes menstrual cycles.

Dong Quai contains coumarins which are very effective in dilating blood vessels, increasing the blood flow in the body and helping in the stimulation of the nervous system. Coumarins reduce menstrual cramps by relaxing the uterus muscles.

Amenorrhea is a condition in which the periods are either missed or are irregular and Dong Quai is used for the treatment of this condition. Dong Quai is also used when they are heavy or prolonged periods. The herb has anti-inflammatory and antispasmodic properties that are responsible for alleviating these conditions.

When Dong Quai is used along with chasteberry, it reduces pain that arises due to endometriosis. Hot flashes that are related to menopause can be controlled if Dong Quai is used with ginseng, chasteberry and black cohosh.

Dong Quai is rich in vitamin B12 and helps the body produce more red blood cells.

Traditional Chinese doctors swore by it to improve circulation of blood in the body and to treat high blood pressure.

Dong Quai is available in different forms like capsules, tinctures, and liquids. It can be bought from health food stores and herbal medicine stores where it is sold as a dried herb. This herb can be used to make a tea that has a soothing and calming effect.

Dong Quai Summary

●Dong Quai is used more among women as it helps improve uterine health, which in turn regularizes menstrual cycles.

●Dong Quai contains coumarins which are very effective in dilating blood vessels, increasing the blood flow in the body and helping in the stimulation of the nervous system. Coumarins reduce menstrual cramps by relaxing the uterus muscles.

●When Dong Quai is used along with chasteberry, it reduces pain that arises due to endometriosis. Hot flashes that are related to menopause can be controlled if Dong Quai is used with ginseng, chasteberry and black cohosh.

●Dong Quai is rich in vitamin B12 and helps the body produce more red blood cells.

PARSLEY

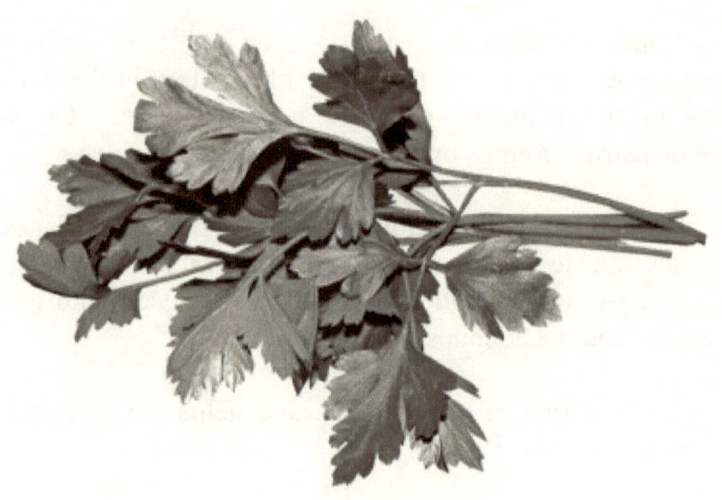

Is parsley something you pick out of a great looking dish at a restaurant and toss to the side of your plate?

I hope not!

That sprig of bright green packs quite a healthy punch and is a lot more than just a decoration for your food. Yes, it is an herb that is full of goodness. Once you know how good it is for you, you'll think twice about casting it aside.

Parsley is for the most part used for its flavor. It has a wonderful fresh flavor that many people enjoy.

It is available all year and you can pick it up at any store. It is a cousin of the other popular herb, celery and is used almost all over the world. It is so easy to grow - all you need to do is plant it once and it is perennial, that is, it keeps growing from the same plant year after year.

People who love the flavor of parsley, and there are many who do, often prefer to grow their own in a pot on the kitchen window or in the herb garden in their backyard.

Let's look at that sprig of parsley again with different eyes. It's a lot more than just a garnish. It's got a couple of very unique compounds and these are responsible for some great health benefits.

One set of parsley compounds is volatile - limonene, eugenol, and myristicin.

The second set is the flavonoids - chrysoeriol, luteolin, apigenin and, apjin.

What do the volatile oils in parsley promise by way of health? Myristicin has been researched and has been proven to reduce the growth of tumors when used on animals.

It is hoped that it does the same with human beings. It is especially good for tumors of the lungs.

The volatile oils in parsley also seem to be a protective force against the damage from cigarette smoke.

So there's a lot more to parsley than garnishes. In fact, parsley that's put into a juicer can be quite a refreshing drink.

There are two main varieties of parsley that you can buy - the Italian flat leaf one and the curly leaf variety. The former has a stronger flavor but is less bitter than the latter.

There is also a third variety of parsley many don't know about called the turnip-rooted parsley. This is grown mainly for its roots.

Whichever type of parsley you choose to buy, make sure it's the freshest you can get. This isn't that difficult considering that most stores stock it all year.

Of course, you can always grow your own parsley and you'll find it's quite easy to do. Then all you need to do when you want a dash of healthy goodness is to reach out and pluck it.

Parsley Summary

•What do the volatile oils in parsley promise by way of health? Myristicin has been researched and has been proved to reduce the growth of tumors when used on animals.

•The volatile oils in parsley also seem to be a protective force against the damage from cigarette smoke.

PEPPERMINT

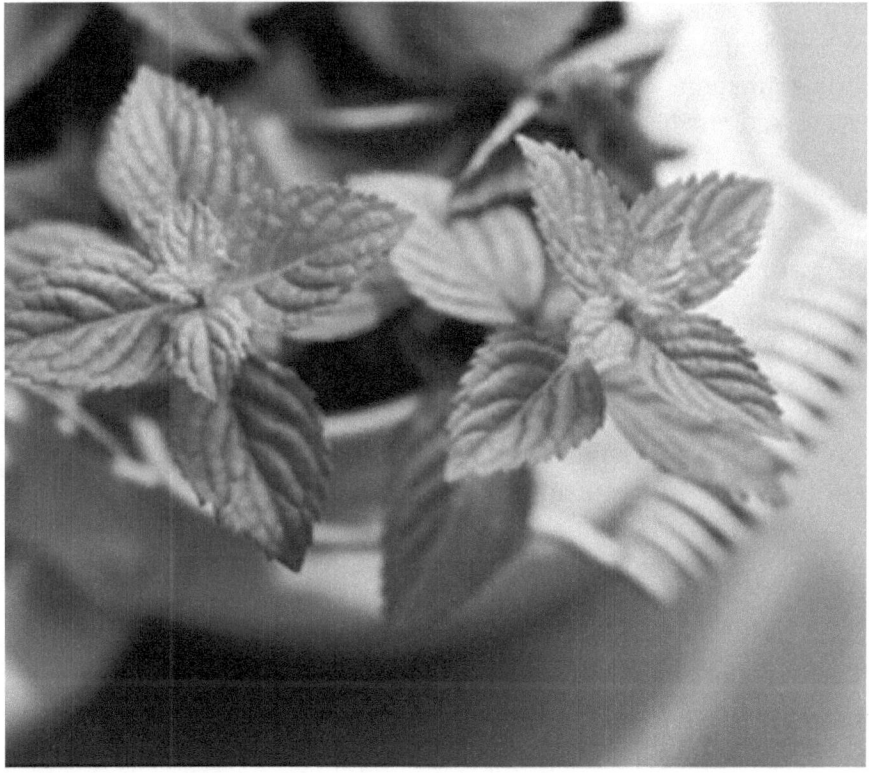

Peppermint is one of the most loved flavors in all the world.

However, peppermint goes beyond just adding zing and zest to your food. Peppermint is also known for its healing powers.

For instance, tea made from peppermint leaves is said to cure minor infections and settle a turbulent stomach. It helps in the digestion of food and eases the digestive tract of irritants.

Those who have sensitive stomachs, and irritable bowels, can find great relief from tea made with fresh peppermint leaves.

Topical peppermint can be used on fungal infections and cuts. Peppermint is also effective in combating allergies and bringing relief to asthma patients.

When you buy peppermint leaves, be mindful of the source. Contamination could be a health hazard. Besides, no two manufacturers have the same quality standards.

Seek out the manufacturer who has an up-to-date manufacturing facility. Sometimes manufacturers tend to over process Peppermint.

Over processing weakens the therapeutic effect of peppermint leaves.

To be sure that the quality of peppermint leaves is good you can cultivate the plant yourself. It is not difficult to grow.

Moreover, the peppermint fragrance adds a lovely scent to your home.

Recipes that can help you reap the maximum benefits from peppermint are aplenty. The most common one is peppermint tea. One method of preparing tea is to put a teaspoon or two of peppermint leaves that have been dried, into a pot.

Set the required quantity of water on the stove but don't allow it to boil. When the water is piping hot, pour it over the peppermint leaves.

Strain the tea and drink it. It's not only the tea that helps but also the aroma while the tea is brewing. So remember to take a deep breath and let the steam and the peppermint aroma do the rest.

Besides soothing the bowels and digestive system, this herbal tea is an antidote for nausea.

If for some reason you don't want to drink peppermint tea, there are always capsules packed with peppermint leaves that you could take instead.

Peppermint is well worth a try. It tastes good, it smells so good, it doesn't feel like medicine at all.

Peppermint Summary

•Tea made from peppermint leaves is said to cure minor infections and settle a turbulent stomach. It helps in the digestion of food and eases the digestive tract of irritants.

•Topical peppermint can be used on fungal infections and cuts. Peppermint is also effective in combating allergies and bringing relief to asthma patients.

PYGEUM

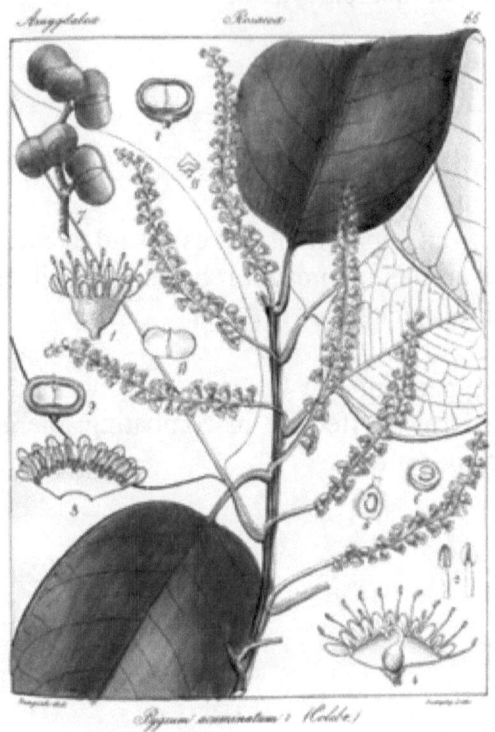

Pygeum acuminatum? (Colebr.)

Just as women suffer from gynecological problems, men have their own problem area - the prostate gland.

There are different kinds of complications that might occur from the malfunctioning of the prostate. Unfortunately, most men go through this difficult experience at some stage in their lives. Consequently, they go in search of remedies that will eradicate or ease their particular symptoms.

There are remedies aplenty but one of the most sensational natural cures available is pygeum.

Pygeum often appears in combination with other compounds like nettle, beta-sitosterol and saw palmetto. You can find these supplements on shelves in the prostate health section of any pharmaceutical store.

Many herbal remedies that cater to problems of the prostate gland, also help swelling subside. Pygeum is one of them.

Pygeum can be bought off the shelf in health food outlets.

Pygeum Summary

•Many herbal remedies that cater to problems of the prostate gland, also help swelling subside. Pygeum is one of them.

SEA BUCKTHORN OIL

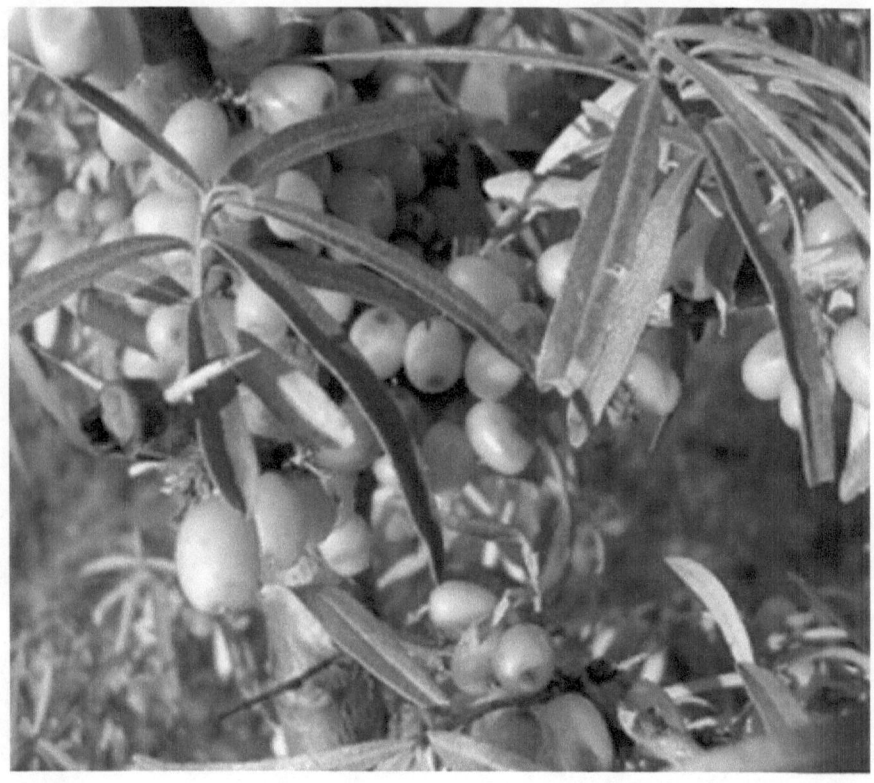

The name is intriguing, the nutritional value is unbelievable.

Sea Buckthorn Oil is one of the latest entrants into the health scene and it is already making waves as an incredible nutritional supplement. Today, there are many studies to help us understand the benefits of Sea Buckthorn Oil.

Sea Buckthorn Oil is from a wild bush that grows in the Gobi desert in the Asian subcontinent. It is an incredibly sturdy and hardy bush, being capable of withstanding extreme temperatures, both heat and cold.

The oil from these plants is at its nutritional best when it is from plants that are harvested from these harsh conditions. Which is why it is of the utmost importance that you know the source of your sea buckthorn oil.

Sea Buckthorn Oil has been used for its medicinal value for centuries by the Mongolian and the Tibetan people.

Over 50 years ago, Russian and Chinese scientists were intrigued by this oil and set about studying the benefits of the bark, the leaves, the seeds, the berries and, the oil.

They tried to measure its efficacy in medicine, nutrition as well as in cosmetics. Today, it has been found that the best parts of the plant to be used to make the oil are the seeds and the berries.

The most valuable product of the plant is the oil and more and more supplements are including it in their formulas.

Sea Buckthorn Oil is rich in vitamin C, vitamin E, beta carotene as well as many flavonoids.

Free radicals tend to damage the cells in the body and the presence of antioxidants is imperative in order to stop them from doing this.

Let's look at what constitutes Sea Buckthorn Oil.

The plant has a minimum of 190 bioactive substances and the oil contains around 106 of these.

Sea Buckthorn Oil is today touted as being a rich source of vitamin E, vitamin C, flavonoids, unsaturated fatty acids, and essential amino acids.

Let's compare it with other supplements.

It has nine times the vitamin E as corn oil, thirty-five times that of soybean oil and nine times that of wheat oil. What's more, 90% of its fatty acids are unsaturated.

Sea Buckthorn Oil is also a wonderful source of omega fatty acids which help make sure that the blood pressure and cholesterol levels in the body stay at the desired levels.

Sea Buckthorn Oil Summary

●Sea Buckthorn Oil is rich in vitamin C, vitamin E, beta carotene as well as many flavonoids.

●Sea Buckthorn Oil is also a wonderful source of omega fatty acids which help make sure that the blood pressure and cholesterol levels in the body stay at the desired levels.

SIBERIAN GINSENG ROOT

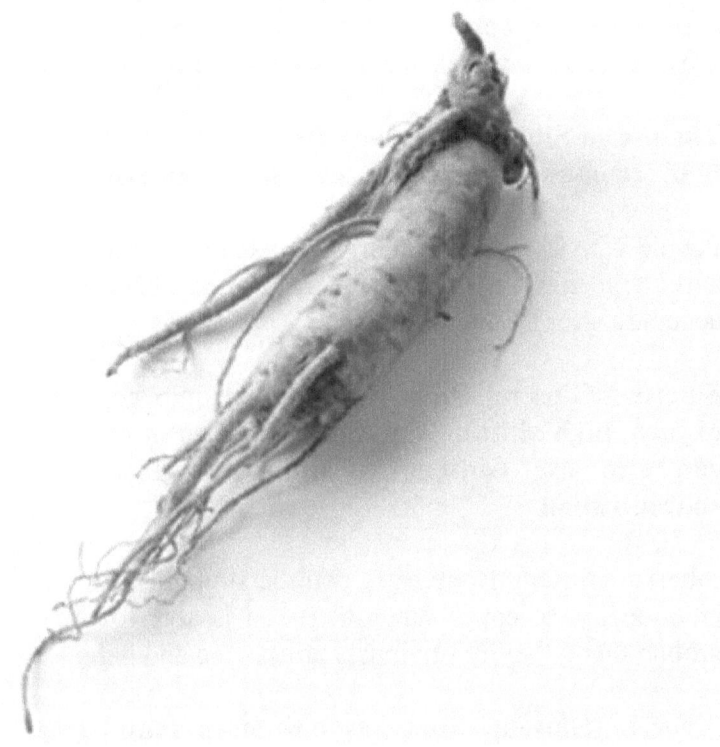

Siberian Ginseng Root, a Chinese secret for thousands of years, gained popularity in the west a few decades ago.

Besides being used as an energy tonic it also has healing and stress-reducing powers.

Siberian Ginseng Root can also be used to enhance memory and to keep flu and colds at bay.

Siberian Ginseng Root is acquiring more and more followers in recent years as its reputation of making a person more vital grows.

The Chinese firmly believed that Siberian Ginseng Root revived the qi or the energy in our bodies and fill us with vitality.

Ginseng's healing properties come from the many unique compounds it contains that have a positive effect on the adrenal glands, which secrete stress-reducing hormones.

The use of Siberian Ginseng Root increases the body's ability to overcome stress and to resist various diseases.

People who have used Siberian Ginseng Root have endorsed this and claim that they could perform better, faster and with greater accuracy after having used it.

Siberian Ginseng Root also helps people cope better in low oxygen, high altitude situations and also in extreme heat. You can also use Ginseng to improve mental alertness and concentration.

Siberian Ginseng Root gives you the strength, both physically and emotionally, to cope. When a person is able to cope with things around them, they're obviously stress-free and happy.

Siberian Ginseng Root has also been found to be effective against fibromyalgia and chronic fatigue syndrome.

Many people have felt increased energy levels after they have taken this Ginseng.

Traditionally, the Chinese used Ginseng as an aphrodisiac and to enhance their fertility levels.

It is believed that Siberian Ginseng Root reduces male impotence and increases the fertility levels in both males as well as females. There is ongoing medical research in trying to prove these claims.

Traditionally, the root has been found effective in treating menopause and it seems to tone up the uterine muscles as well as stabilize hormone levels. So it also helps relieve menstrual cramps.

You can buy Siberian Ginseng Root over the Internet or at health stores, and Asian supermarkets.

Siberian Ginseng Root Summary

●Siberian Ginseng Root can also be used to enhance memory and to keep flu and colds at bay.

●Ginseng's healing properties come from the many unique compounds it contains that have a positive effect on the adrenal glands, which secrete stress-reducing hormones.

●Siberian Ginseng Root increases the body's ability to overcome stress and to resist various diseases.

●Siberian Ginseng Root helps people cope better in low oxygen, high altitude situations and also in extreme heat. You can also use Ginseng to improve mental alertness and concentration.

●Siberian Ginseng Root has also been found to be effective against fibromyalgia and chronic fatigue syndrome.

●It is believed that Siberian Ginseng Root reduces male impotence and increases the fertility levels in both males as well as females. There is ongoing medical research in trying to prove these claims.

●Siberian Ginseng Root has been found effective in treating menopause and it seems to tone up the uterine muscles as well as stabilize hormone levels. So it also helps relieve menstrual cramps.

STRAWBERRIES

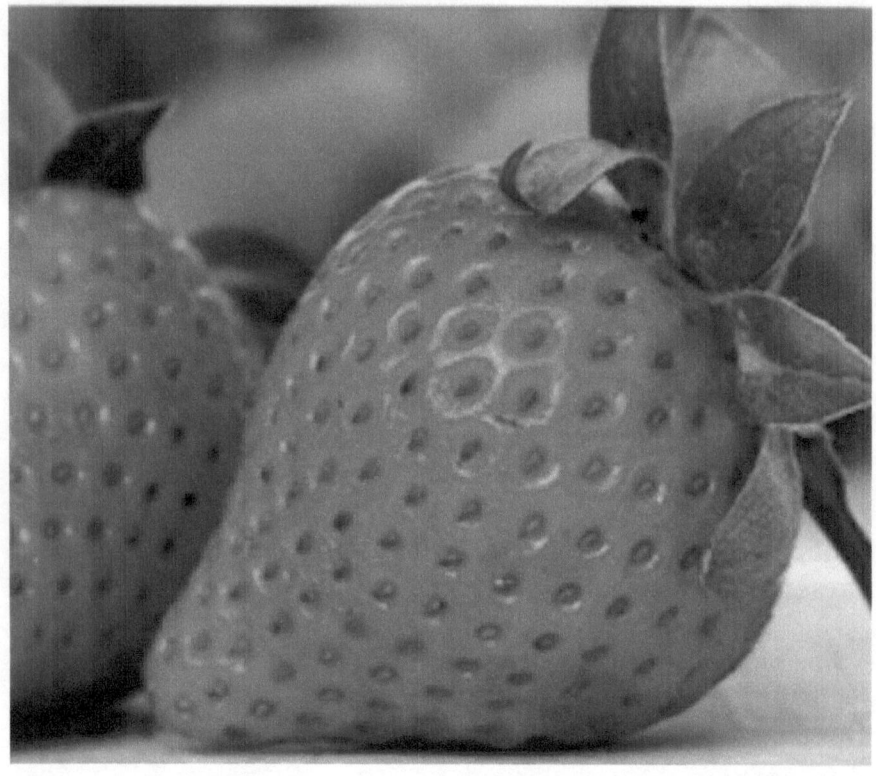

Almost everybody who has eaten strawberries will agree that this fruit is absolutely delicious.

An added bonus comes in knowing that strawberries are as nutritious as they are delicious. Not many foods give you this irresistible combination, so you could indulge in strawberries frequently without feeling guilty.

The recommended daily dose of vegetables and fresh fruits is a minimum of five servings but in reality, far too many people do not eat enough of fruit and vegetables.

Fresh strawberries can be added to your daily menu in a variety of ways. They can be used in fruit salads, in oatmeal, or just on their own.

Let's look at strawberries nutritional value. Strawberries are loaded with the goodness of Vitamin C.

They also contain very high levels of antioxidants, phytonutrients, and many other nutrients.

Antioxidants have been proven to reduce the damage caused by free radicals and are an important part of any diet.

This little fruit is packed with nutrients including folic acid, vitamin K, riboflavin, omega-3 fatty acids, manganese, copper, vitamin B6, potassium, magnesium and vitamin B5.

Strawberries are in demand all year round because of the great taste. Unfortunately, this fruit is very delicate and great care has to taken while transporting and storing them. Strawberries do not last long once they are picked and you have to buy only what you need for a few days at a time.

At times when fresh strawberries are not available, you can make do with frozen strawberries.

It is important to remember that strawberries do not ripen after they are picked. So choose the reddest, ripest strawberries as these will be the tastiest and have the highest amount of nutrients. Make sure that the strawberries you choose are firm and unbruised.

Contrary to popular opinion, medium strawberries sometimes taste sweeter than the larger sized ones.

Being such delicate fruits, strawberries should be handled very carefully. Do not pack them very tightly as they would get crushed and damaged. Separate any strawberries that show signs of mold as this could spread and contaminate the whole lot.

Strawberries can be stored in the refrigerator for a few days in a bowl covered by a plastic wrap.

Strawberries Summary

●This little fruit is packed with nutrients including folic acid, vitamin K, riboflavin, omega-3 fatty acids, manganese, copper, vitamin B6, potassium, magnesium and vitamin B5.

VALERIAN ROOT

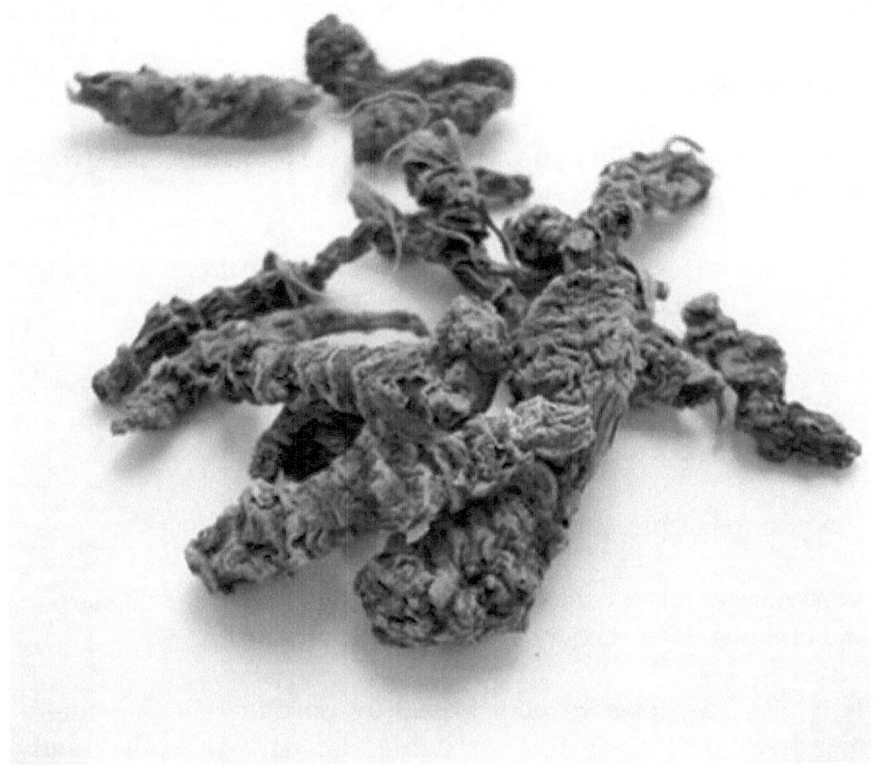

There are people in this world who can sleep almost standing up, whenever they want, and wherever they want.

Then there are people who are not able to sleep at all.

They have to resort to pills and other solutions to catch some shut-eye or they will not be able to function efficiently. We call this insomnia.

Insomnia is a huge problem and it responsible for a lot of anguish, health problems, and loss of productivity in the world.

Valerian root is a natural solution for insomnia.

Found growing wild in many places all over the globe Valerian root has proven its usefulness for many centuries now.

It is a perennial herb and is non-addictive.

Valerian root is mild and works well to treat anxiety and stress too.

This plant has stems and roots underground which are dried and converted into herbal preparations.

It is important to note that post-harvest handling is a delicate issue. If the machinery used is not of the best quality, the effectiveness of Valerian root can be reduced.

Valerian root capsules are what most people prefer using.

Valerian root relaxes tense muscles so it's good for relieving stress and bringing down anxiety and even panic attacks.

It is also suspected to play a healthy part in relieving some digestive problems like irritable bowel syndrome and diverticulosis.

The root is seen to have a soothing effect irrespective of the form of consumption. It could be tablets, capsules, powder, herbal tea or as an essential oil.

Valerian Root Summary

• Valerian root is a natural solution for insomnia.

●Valerian root is mild and works well to treat anxiety and stress too.

●Valerian root is also suspected to play a healthy part in relieving some digestive problems like irritable bowel syndrome and diverticulosis.

PART 2

How To Achieve Specific Health Goals With Superfoods

KEEP YOUR YOUTH WITH SUPERFOODS

Let's face it; we all want to look fresh and vibrant.

We end up spending a ridiculous amount of money lathering up our faces with lotions made from some rare sea-cucumber to little or no avail.

Or, we saddle up on the doctor's seat for expensive shots and after one too many our friends begin to ask us what's wrong; why do we always have that frozen, semi-startled look on our faces.

Isn't there a better way to the fountain of youth?

That's where Superfoods come in!

Mother Nature has always wanted us to look our very best and in her infinite wisdom - not only did she create a group of foods that can help us hang on to the rosy glow of our youth, she's actually made it quite simple - she color coded it!

In the league of Superfoods, it's the color of the food that can help you understand how to put together a balanced diet that will help you look like a perky co-ed on the outside and help you feel like a triathlete on the inside!

Follow these easy steps to stay looking young:

Purple, Blue, Red keeps you young on the inside - When you see fruits with these colors they most likely have loads of a pigment called anthocyanins - which are part of the flavonoid family of antioxidants that will keep your body young from in the inside out.

There was a recent study that demonstrated their ability to actually "turn off" a set of genes that are responsible for causing the cells in our body to "naturally" die.

They literally slow the dying process in our body. Not only that, they also prevent inflammation. Anthocyanins are found heavily concentrated in berries; acai berries (blackish-purple), blueberries, cranberries, and all other berries. The darker the color of the berry the more anthocyanin it contains.

Orange and Green make your skin and hair pretty - Orange foods like pumpkin, acorn squash, carrots, sweet potatoes are orange because they have phytonutrients called **carotenes.**

These Superfoods are the youth bomb, loaded with both alpha and beta carotenes, once these nutrients go into your body, your liver converts it to Vitamin A.

And here's the bonus, if the liver doesn't need all the Vitamin A, it will store it and not flush it out!

Vitamin A is the magic elixir that reverses the effects of sun damage on your skin. It also replaces the sebum in your scalp which gives your hair a lustrous, healthy gloss and prevents it from looking dry and frizzy.

Spinach, broccoli, and cabbages are additional sources of Vitamin A. They are green because of heavy concentrations of chlorophyll which is another powerful group of phytonutrients.

As an added benefit, in many greens are a group of polysaccharides that give a mega-boost to the immune system. Like the anthocyanins, the darker the color the more of a powerhouse it will be in terms of benefiting your body.

Brown keeps your skin glowing - Nuts, in all shapes and sizes (and usually brown) are loaded with Omega 3 oils that keep your skin moist and plump.

This is earth's natural lotion that helps the skin lock in water and in conjunction with Vitamin A gives your skin a radiant quality. You can also get a healthy dose of Omega 3's from fish oil, and flaxseed oil.

So, you have the list and now you know the colors to paint a more youthful you, so skip the beauty aisle and head for the fruit and produce section the next time you go shopping!

LOSING WEIGHT WITH SUPER FOODS

Counting calories, keeping track of color cards, waiting for the postman to come with your next meal in a box, we've all suffered through the rigors of a weight loss program - and for what - to show off the five pounds we lost that nobody seems to notice?

Why is there so much work involved in losing so little weight?

Weight loss doesn't have to be a ritual if we understand how our bodies work and knowing which foods offer the most power.

Luckily, Superfoods are the high octane fuel that our body needs.

They're incredible for raising your metabolism while reducing the insulin in your body.

This combination gives you more energy throughout the day without feeling like a famine victim.

In other words, once you go Superfoods, you don't go back to playing the weight-loss circuit. *Let's cut our losses for good!*

There are three concepts you need to know in order to sustain an ideal weight with a healthy metabolism.

The first is how frequently you eat. Research proves that it's better to eat six mini-meals a day versus three large ones. This is critical to keeping your metabolism running at a balanced rate.

The second involves how much you eat, if you think starving yourself will help you lose weight, you're wrong. It does the opposite.

Eating less than 1,000 calories a day will spook your basal metabolism. It will basically operate on slow-to-stop mode until you prove to it you're not in a famine so, eat up - just be healthy about it!

The third is quality over quantity, and that's where Superfoods come into play!

Grapefruit; Researchers have found that not only is this fruit rich in Vitamin C and limonoids (cancer-fighting agents) it inhibits the amount of insulin your body produces when you eat and will give you that stuffed feeling.

Oatmeal + Berries + Cinnamon; Equals perfect breakfast meal. The oatmeal reduces your cholesterol, the berries are antioxidants and the cinnamon will reduce insulin levels.

Cinnamon is a secret weapon in the fight against weight loss and diabetes type II. In one study, they found that about half a teaspoon of cinnamon is enough to reduce your blood-insulin level by almost half. This means you won't feel hunger pains and cravings as frequently!

Super Fruits; Apples, pears, and oranges are great for mini-meal snacks. They have fructose which is a natural sugar that the body breaks down fast and keeps it fueled. Also, apples and pears have pectin fiber which is excellent for reducing blood-insulin levels.

Pumpkin - Is there no end to all that pumpkin does for the body? Pumpkin is loaded with fiber which is critical for expelling toxins and waste which keeps your metabolism in peak condition. Not to mention, pumpkin is packed with tons of nutrients that are good for your skin, your hair and even your liver.

Sardines- Can you believe that these little fishies can help you look fit and trim? They are crammed with high levels of protein and Omega 3's both of which are a 1-2 punch that will boost your metabolism and keep your heart ready for all the exercise you should be doing with a healthy diet! Don't fret about the taste, if you lightly sauté the sardines, they'll take on the flavor profile of roasted nuts. Yum!

Green Tea- This is your insurance clause to keeping your metabolism running at optimum speed. If you drink 8 glasses of water a day, why not throw in a green tea bag? This guarantees, even if you don't eat other Superfoods, to still kick your metabolism into high gear. Green tea also has loads of catechins which are antioxidants that help your immune system.

Healthy eating tips:

Our grandparents ate well balanced healthy meals and they had healthier lives. In today's time-conscious, fast-paced, urban lifestyle, quick convenient meals have become the norm.

Scientific studies have shown that diet is the most important factor for a long, healthy life. Many common disorders and diseases can be avoided by improving the daily diet.

Eat healthy by getting rid of processed foods and eating more foods with high fiber content, like fresh fruits, vegetables, grains, and legumes.

The FDA's new guidelines recommend five servings of fruit and vegetables.

A great variety of fresh produce is available all year round. Fruits and vegetables are important sources of vitamins and antioxidants in addition to soluble fibers that help eliminate the toxins and waste products from our bodies.

Eat a good mixture of green, yellow, orange and red-purple fruits and vegetables. Eating a wide variety of foods is important for the daily intake of proteins, carbohydrates, vitamins, and minerals.

Meat is good but it is best to eat lean meats with all the fat trimmed off.

Avoid processed meats as they are high in fats and salts.

Fish is a great source of protein and has good, heart-protecting omega-3 fatty acids. Two to three portions of fish a week will really help lower cholesterol and improve the skin tone. Nuts too provide both nutrition and healthy fats.

It is very important to use the right cooking oil. Oils add fats and lots of calories and it's best not to use oils with unhealthy saturated fats. Oils containing polyunsaturated fats like olive oil are cardiovascular protectors. Do not use lard.

Whole grain foods like whole wheat bread are better and have a greater mineral, vitamin and fiber content than highly processed white bread.

Beans and legumes provide good carbohydrates and are nutritious.

Take into consideration your current state of health with a checkup which includes blood pressure, cholesterol, and other routine blood and urine tests.

This will give you a base to start from. A regular physical once a year along with healthy eating could save your life.

Healthy eating is a choice. It does not have to be boring or bland.

An occasional burger will not harm you. Eat a healthy balanced diet filled with Superfoods and you will feel better. That's all it takes.

Recipes and books are available on how to make healthy dishes. So the next time you are grocery shopping, stop and think what's good for you.

PROTECT YOURSELF FROM CANCER WITH SUPERFOODS

The good news is that cancer is no longer the death sentence it once was. The bad news, chemotherapy isn't exactly a day at Disneyland. In fact, a lot of survivors will tell you that it's the next to worst thing to actually suffering from cancer.

Well, the even better news is that, thankfully, we have some of the smartest minds on the planet looking for cures that will not just defeat cancer but also help prevent us from ever having to be told we have it.

And what many of these researchers have discovered is that Mother Nature is working alongside to help us!

Broccoli - Eating lots of it might just prevent you from ever having to step into a chemotherapy treatment center. Evidence is pouring in about its ability to work with our body to destroy the essential building blocks of not just one or two cancers, but many cancers.

Who knew, the Rudolph of the food world, dreaded by most eaters, is now being hailed as one of the most powerful foods on Earth!

Broccoli contains a megadose of a nutrient called sulforaphane that in turn triggers the body's natural production of type II enzymes. The sulforaphane causes the body to produce armies and armies of this enzyme that flood the body looking for cancerous, mutant cells.

This is key because these type II enzymes are the natural killers of cancer cells - and the best defense against developing cancer. Nobody's been able to explain why this relationship exists, but for whatever reasons, type II enzymes have it hot for sulforaphane, and broccoli's got the motherload of it.

Broccoli also has another phytonutrient called isothiocyanates that also helps stop cancer in its tracks, especially noticeable in lung and stomach cancers.

And if that weren't enough, broccoli is also packing another punch with indoles, another compound that was discovered to cut off certain estrogen based compounds that are needed for tumors to grow.

So, not only does broccoli help prevent cancer, it can actually attack the cancerous formations that have developed in your body. That's one dedicated vegetable!

Berries - Purple, blue and red ones - eat them all! Those anthocyanins are at again! It seems there's nothing these little antioxidants can't do!

These guys along with the ellagic acids and pterostilbene that are also found in berries do a 1-2-3 triple threat on cancer formation and growth.

Evidence, like with broccoli, is showing that it's effective on the root level of most cancers, having a demonstrable effect on all sorts from esophageal to lung and liver cancers.

Tomatoes and Watermelons - both have lycopene, which by now as many of you know, has become the poster child antioxidant in stopping cancer.

And it deserves the credit.

Lycopene is a powerful agent in helping stop the growth of prostate cancer. Not only that, lycopene is also showing significant promise in helping with cardiovascular diseases.

So, if you find tomatoes a little bitter, watermelon is a very good alternative as it has a heavier concentration of both lycopene and Vitamin C.

It's wonderful that we live in a world where we can receive treatments for our illnesses so that we can stay healthy.

But what's even more wonderful is that staying healthy is as easy as making Superfoods part of our daily diets!

SUPERFOODS FOR A SHARP MIND

Did you forget where you put the cars keys again? Or worse, did you forget that person's name again even though they already told you twice before?

Between our cell phones and computers we now have to remember more information than ever and having to recall it at a moment's notice. *How do we survive information overload?*

Diet. Yes, diet is a powerful and direct way that we can affect the architecture that controls memory and cognition. There are a couple of things to remember when finding foods that will boost your brain power.

You want foods that will help your blood - because oxygen-rich blood is the power source for the brain. Second, you want foods that will nurture your nervous system because it's the electrical wiring that processes brain activity.

Here's a list of some of the best foods that address the needs, and who knows, may just make you the genius you need to be to function in this wireless world of information!

Berries - Hopefully when you hear this word you will think more of the fruity kind that you eat and less of the kind that you diddle with your fingers. Berries are the powerhouse of brain power. They are especially concentrated with anthocyanins, epicatechins, and resveratrol, all of which are especially powerful in improving cellular function in all parts of the body, but especially the brain and heart. The darker the berry the more power it contains.

In general, if you don't prefer berries try some apples, oranges, or anything green. They also have tons of phytonutrients like Vitamin C which is excellent at oxidizing toxic fat—a known contributor to Alzheimer's. Not to mention, all fruits and vegetables are loaded with fiber which is good for overall general health.

Fish - Also known as the miracle meat. Fish like Salmon, Sardines, Bluefish, Herring, Mackerel and Tuna are good for both the heart and the brain because of their rich supply of Omega-3 fatty acids.

Omega 3 is an essential fatty acid that the body cannot produce but requires to live and is vital to brain function. Researchers are discovering that having it consistently can even temper behavioral problems like bipolar disorder and ADHD.

Sardines are especially important because they are small and are not as riddled with mercury and other ocean pollutants as bigger fish which have higher concentrations.

And no, you do not have to make a special trip to the fishmonger; buying the canned variety will also give you the nutrition you need.

If you don't like fish, you can also eat nuts and plant-based oils which also have vital fatty acids.

Vitamin B- Vitamin B12 and B6 are critical to protecting the nervous system of the body and this, of course, includes the brain. Spinach, leafy greens and broccoli contain loads of it, so does orange vegetables like carrots and pumpkin. Seeds and nuts are also rich in Vitamin B. If you eat meat, poultry including eggs are rich sources of it as are dairy products.

Short of having Intel drive over and install memory chips in our brain, there's only one real option that we have to improve our brain power and memory - a better diet and exercise program.

Better eating means better living - and a decent memory to boot!

THE POWER OF GREEN SUPERFOODS

Let's be honest, in the world of Superfoods, nobody will accuse these leafy greens as being *fabulous*.

They may not be as glamorous as a salmon fillet served at a five star restaurant, and they may not be as sweet and delicious as blueberries frolicking in whipped cream, nor will they ever be as popular as pumpkin is in the Fall - but leafy greens will keep you alive, and make you feel great about yourself.

Leafy greens are the modest Superfoods.

They eschew the glitz and glamour and just want to help improve the lives of all who consume them. In fact, most leafy greens are some of the best sources of Vitamin E, which is critical in slowing down the decline of mental ability. Not only that, they get along with all other foods - when can't you serve a salad with a meal?

When can't you have a side of greens with a dish?

Eating these guys in steady supply will make you feel alive!

Spinach - Sure it got a bad rap with that E. Coli poisoning in 2006, and maybe Popeye the Sailorman wasn't the best spokesperson, but don't write it off - PR was never a strong suit of Spinach!

And thankfully, Popeye has moved on to Fried Chicken.

Intensive research is underway with spinach because, like broccoli, researchers keep finding all of these amazing things it can do!

It's loaded with Vitamin C and A, and they work together to prevent the cholesterol in your body from oxidizing, which prevents it from solidifying - so, it reduces damage and obstruction of your blood vessels.

Overall, spinach is a known Superfood that promotes a healthy cardiovascular system.

Spinach also has 13 confirmed antioxidants that researchers are demonstrating can prevent and treat prostate cancer, ovarian cancer, and can even prevent macular degeneration. So you see, your grandmother was right after all, eating spinach can improve your eyesight.

Last but not least, spinach is a mega-dose source of Folic Acid and that all pregnant women need for a healthy strong baby, and that the rest of us need for all sorts of things from strong bones, to well running gastrointestinal health.

Spirulina - Yummy, who wants to nibble on some green/blue algae!? Just kidding, spirulina (thankfully) comes in powder or tablet form and should definitely be consumed - especially if you're vegetarian.

There's still a lot of debate about the true benefits of spirulina but what most everyone can agree on is that spirulina is an excellent and expensive source of protein, along with 8 critical amino acids our bodies need. Not only that, but it also has GLA, an essential fatty acid.

The promise of spirulina is still unfolding, but if it proves to be true - it may be known as an HIV killer and also a way to reduce allergies and inflammations. But the research on these findings is still preliminary.

Grasses- Again, not to suggest that we chew the cud, but wheat grass and barley grass are very important sources of chlorophyll, a phytonutrient that can beat up cancer and give you boosts of energy. They also contain a protein called P4D1 which has powerful anti-inflammatory properties.

Most people who use the fresh variety, only use the baby growth and process it into their juicers with other products like carrots. Or, you can also buy the powder form and mix it into a shake. Either way, eating these grasses can improve your overall health.

HELPING THE ENVIRONMENT WITH PLANT-BASED SUPERFOODS

Global warming is a topic of serious discussion in homes, coffee shops, late-night television, and governmental committee meetings.

The problem with these discussions is that there seems to be very little an individual person can do to help solve the problem with the possible exception of finding alternative transportation on a daily basis either in the form of walking more, riding a bike, using public transportation or investing in one of the newer vehicles that emits a greatly reduced amount of carbon dioxide.

Attention has recently been directed at the animal agriculture industry, especially in the United States.

The United Nations reported that raising animals for their meat generates more greenhouse gases in the form of methane and nitrous oxide than all the cars and trucks in the world emit in the form of carbon dioxide gas.

Global warming is a direct result of the emission of three greenhouse gases; carbon dioxide, methane, and nitrous oxide. Carbon dioxide is the direct result of burning fossil fuels. Methane and nitrous oxide are a direct result of farming animals for their meat.

The best news in the face of these dire warnings is that each individual now has the power to make a direct contribution to lessening the production of greenhouse gases.

Plant-based Superfoods diets have been proven to emit far fewer greenhouse gases than any other type of diet in use today.
Raising animals causes not only global warming, but it increases air and water pollution, water shortages, degradation of farmable land, and ignores the importance of biodiversity in the use of our farmland.

It has been proven that the amount of vegetable food raised for animal agriculture is four times what it would take to feed humans as end consumers of the vegetable products.
The United States specifically is responsible for over one-quarter of the world's ever-increasing greenhouse emissions. Over 1.5 tons are directly attributed to American's insatiable taste for meat, whether it is beef, lamb, and poultry. The idea is not necessarily to convert everyone to vegetarianism but to cut down on our meat consumption.

Two direct benefits to this action would be improved health of the American people, and a healthier planet due to decreased greenhouse gases.
Per capita, American consumption of meat has increased in the past 50 years. The surprising correlation to increased heart disease is not to be ignored. Increased meat consumption has increased the intake of dietary trans-fats found in the meat we consume.

Increased meat consumption has led to an unhealthy American population and an unhealthy earth environment. A true vegetarian diet is the only diet proven by Dr. Dean Ornish to halt and even reverse the course of cardiac disease. The only other way to achieve this sort of success is through the use of numerous and very expensive drugs.
Decreasing methane and nitrous oxide producers by turning toward a diet that is based on Plant-based Superfoods is easier to accomplish than all our past efforts to decrease carbon dioxide emissions.

We can make a bigger impact on the environment by turning to a Plant-based Superfoods diet than by buying a hybrid vehicle for transportation. In addition to eating a vegetarian diet, it is a good idea to look for vegan-certified personal care products for a well-rounded approach to helping to save our world.

STAYING HEALTHY WITH SUPERFOODS

All recent talk about Superfoods can be confusing. Which foods are the best?

What if I don't like a Superfood, does that mean I should just give up and return to my readily available fast food meals?

The answer is a resounding "No!"

All Superfoods are good, and each food represents a category of foods that are related and confer upon the consumer similar benefits. The best Superfoods are the ones that you learn to enjoy and eat on a daily or weekly basis.

The following is a list comprised of a dozen Superfoods, but it is just a starting point. Science is discovering new benefits to some of the foods we eat on a regular basis and as a result, the list will continue to grow.

●Whole grains – oats, barley, buckwheat, wheat, brown rice, rye, millet, bulgur, yellow corn, and couscous. 5 – 7 servings per day.

●Nuts and Seeds – Walnuts, almonds peanuts, pinon, pecan, sunflower and pumpkin seeds. 1 ounce five times per week.

●Fish – Wild Alaskan salmon (fresh or canned), halibut, herring, albacore tuna, trout, sardines, oysters and clams. 2 – 4 times per week.

●Dark Greens – Spinach, kale, chard, broccoli, brussel sprouts, sprouts of all kinds. 1 – 2 cups per day.

- Beans – Pinto, green, black, kidney, peas, garbanzo, Navy, Great Northern. Four 1/2 –cup servings per week.

- Berries – Blueberries, blackberries, raspberries, cranberries, goji berries. 1 – 2 cups per day.

- Citrus – Oranges, mandarins, grapefruit, lemon, lime, kumquat, tangerines. 1 serving per day.

- Orange Vegetables – Pumpkin, butternut squash. ½ cup per day.

- Turkey breast – skinless, cooked without added fat. 3 – 4 servings per week.

- Yogurt – live-cultured, unsweetened. 2 cups per day.

- Tea – Black, green, white.

Whole Grains have a myriad of health benefits, so if you want your bread and eat it too, be certain that the first ingredient is some form of whole grain.

Whole grain contains all three parts of the grain, the bran, the endosperm (middle layer), and the germ (inner layer) that is packed full of Vitamin B, E, and other phytochemicals. Oats and barley are especially noted for their cholesterol-lowering abilities. All whole grains are fiber-rich foods that help to control appetite and blood sugar fluctuations.

Nuts and Seeds are good for your heart. They contain heart-healthy protein, fat, vitamins, minerals and many other phytochemicals that fight both heart disease as well as cancer.

Fish, especially cold-water fish are very rich sources of Omega-3 fatty acids that prevent inflammation that can cause heart disease, arthritis, asthma, insulin resistance, ADD and depression. Most Americans are dangerously deficient in Omega-3 fatty acids.

Dark Greens – Eating these veggies can prevent or reverse the advance of cancer, minimize the incidence of birth defects, reduce the risk of cataracts and age-related macular degeneration, improve bone and cardiac health.

Beans – (this category includes both green and dried.) Excellent source of low fat, inexpensive protein that reduces cholesterol, battles heart disease, fights obesity and Type II diabetes by stabilizing blood sugar fluctuations, lowers blood pressure and decreases the incidence of colon problems.

Berries – Blueberries are especially known for their tremendous quantities of disease-fighting antioxidants and are sometimes called brain berries, or youth berries because of their anti-aging characteristics. All berries are full of polyphenols that are nearly miraculous. Go ahead, pile on the blueberry preserves or blackberry jam. It is good for you.

Citrus – Long touted as the first health food due to its high vitamin C content, we might be overlooking the true health benefits of citrus. They fight heart disease, cancer, diabetes, and other chronic illnesses. Enjoy as a whole food or full pulp juice.

Orange Vegetables – Much has been published about the wonders of beta-carotene found in orange vegetables, but new studies have revealed that the alpha-carotene, especially in pumpkin make it one of the most nutritionally valuable foods known because of its ability to reverse signs of aging.

Turkey Breast – Highly nutritious, low fat, and inexpensive. This is the leanest meat protein available today, mimicking the healthiest diets such as Paleolithic, Mediterranean, and Japanese, which have proven that the leaner the protein the better. Good for the heart and immune system.

Yogurt – Posses immune stimulating components in its live cultures, promoting the growth of good GI bacteria while inhibiting the reproduction of bad bacteria. A healthy GI tract = good health throughout the entire body.

Tea – Lowers blood pressure, prevents osteoporosis, and skin cancer, fights wrinkles, is an antiviral, anti-allergy, anti-inflammatory, and prevents cataracts. What else do you want? Tea does it all!

FINAL THOUGHTS

You Want Your Superfoods To Be Organic

In its purest form, organic is about eating food that has not been altered in any way with chemicals that are not part of the natural growth cycle of the food being eaten.

So, when you add high nitrogen-based fertilizer to a crop or split open a hydrogen compound in vegetable oil, or eat meat from cows or chickens that have been inoculated with antibiotics and hormones, you are not eating organic food.

Advocates for organic food argue that the human body has thousands of years of experience in its DNA to break down fruits, vegetable and meats in their natural state absent of additives.

The body simply doesn't know what to do with synthetically created compounds or excessive amounts of chemicals and hormones that are put into foods.

The body goes into Code Red trying to purge these unfamiliar modified chemicals from the body or it stores it in the fat where eventually it can become carcinogenic or cancer-causing. Partially hydrogenated oil or trans fat, which is a chemically modified oil and a cause of cancer illustrates this example.

For decades research and advocacy have pointed to the dangers of producing food that is not organic because of the adverse effects these processes have on the entire ecology of a local environment.

Environmentalists point out that the soil treated full of nitrogen compounds and pesticides eventually washes into local waterways, poisoning the local environment, including the people who rely on local sources of water for consumption, not to mention any aquatic life that people eat.

Nutritionists and physicians are deeply concerned about the long term effects of eating foods that have been treated with pesticides and/or processed with artificial preservatives.

Aside from an explosion of obesity rates in children (largely from preservative rich foods), experts have pointed out that many children are now experiencing an accelerated adolescence that may be the result of ingesting hormone-treated meat (and milk) that is possibly making their bodies undergo pubescence at ages well below the traditional age of twelve and thirteen.

Researchers have no idea what the long term implications of this accelerated aging process will be on this generation of children.

ORGANIC FOOD ORGANIZATIONS

One of the best ways of knowing where to find authentic organic food is to consult organizations who are dedicated to educating consumers about the issue. **Organic Consumers** (http://www.organicconsumers.org/) is a great place to start with understanding the fundamentals of "organic."

Also, **the National Organic Program (NOP)** (http://www.ams.usda.gov/nop/indexIE.htm), which is an entity regulated by the USDA has information on what it considers "organic" along with other interesting information.

It's important to cross-compare their definition with an organization like Organic Consumers because NOP definitions and standards are heavily influenced by powerful food producing corporations who lobby for different standards of "organic" than what consumer advocates consider "organic."

The whole concept has become extremely political, largely because huge food producing corporations have much to lose by not being able to influence the definition of "organic."

So, it's important to educate yourself and understand who is calling what "organic" and what they mean when they use that label.

But one thing is for certain, there is not one person who will argue that eating organic is NOT healthy. Sadly, the same cannot be unequivocally said for eating non-organic.